SPECIALIST MENTAL HEALTHCARE FOR CHILDREN AND ADOLESCENTS

A need for comprehensive services for young people requiring more intensive mental health services has been identified and this book explores what works in Child and Adolescent Mental Health (CAMHS) at this level.

Specialist Mental Healthcare for Children and Adolescents looks at intensive outpatient and community services; assertive outreach teams; inpatient residential and secure provision; and other highly specialised assessment, consultation and intervention services. Based on the best available evidence, each chapter provides key points, research summaries and an overview of available treatments. It outlines emerging good practice guidance, service models, assessment, and training and workforce development requirements.

This accessible text is essential reading for commissioners and professionals – including psychiatrists, psychologists, nurses, therapists, social workers and teachers – working in specialist CAMHS services, as well as all those studying for qualifications in child and adolescent mental health.

Tim McDougall is Nurse Consultant and a Clinical Director at the Cheshire and Wirral NHS Foundation Trust, UK. He is currently Chair of the UK Nurse Consultants in CAMHS Forum and the Quality Network for Inpatient CAMHS (QNIC) Executive Committee.

Andy Cotgrove is a Consultant Adolescent Psychiatrist and Medical Director for Cheshire and Wirral Partnership NHS Foundation Trust, UK.

SPECIALIST MENTAL HEALTHCARE FOR CHILDREN AND ADOLESCENTS

Hospital, intensive community and home-based services

Edited by Tim McDougall and Andy Cotgrove

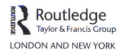

LONDON AND NEW YORK

First published 2014
by Routledge
2 Park Square, Milton Park, Abingdon, Oxon, OX14 4RN

and by Routledge
711 Third Avenue, New York, NY 10017

Routledge is an imprint of the Taylor & Francis Group, an informa business

Note
The views and opinions expressed in this book are those of the
individual chapter authors who are experts in their field.

British Library Cataloguing in Publication Data
A catalogue record for this book is available from the British Library

Library of Congress Cataloging in Publication Data
Specialist mental healthcare for children and adolescents : hospital,
intensive community, and home-based services / edited by Tim
McDougall and Andy Cotgrove.
       p. ; cm.
    Includes bibliographical references.
    I. McDougall, Tim, editor of compilation. II. Cotgrove, Andy, editor
of compilation.
    [DNLM: 1. Mental Health Services – Great Britain. 2. Adolescent –
Great Britain. 3. Adolescent Psychology –methods – Great Britain.
4. Child – Great Britain. 5. Child Psychology – methods –
Great Britain. 6. Needs Assessment – Great Britain. WM 30 FA1]
RA790.7.G7

ISBN: 978-0-415-52090-4 (hbk)
ISBN: 978-0-415-52091-1 (pbk)
ISBN: 978-1-315-85750-3 (ebk)

Typeset in Bembo
by HWA Text and Data Management, London

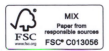

Printed and bound in Great Britain by
TJ International Ltd, Padstow, Cornwall

CONTENTS

ILLUSTRATIONS

Figures

Tables

Boxes

CONTRIBUTORS

Toby Biggins is a Consultant Family Psychotherapist and Service Lead for a Home-based Therapy Service provided by Cheshire and Wirral NHS Foundation Trust. Previously, he developed and led the ROSTA Project – the UK's first treatment foster care service – after a career spent mostly in the USA, where he worked in a number of complex needs CAMHS services in parallel with holding academic positions in the Philadelphia area.

Andy Cotgrove is a Consultant Adolescent Psychiatrist and Medical Director for Cheshire and Wirral Partnership NHS Foundation Trust. Andy qualified from Sheffield Medical School in 1982 and worked in hospital medicine and general practice before training in psychiatry. His specialist training in child and adolescent psychiatry was at the Tavistock Clinic in London where he also gained an MSc in family therapy. Andy has a special interest in service development and improvement, and has led a number of service redesign initiatives within Tier 4 CAMHS. His research and writing has focused on self-harm, use of antidepressants and the role of Tier 4 CAMHS. Over the last 10 years Andy has worked with NICE as a member or advisor to the following NICE Guideline Development Groups: Depression in Young People, Self Harm, Borderline Personality Disorder and Psychosis with Substance Misuse. He was also a long-standing member of the NICE Mental Health Topic Selection Panel and member of the Commissioning Outcomes Framework advisory group. Andy was a clinical director in CAMHS for 17 years before being appointed as a medical director in 2010.

Marie Crofts is the Associate Director for CAMHS at Birmingham Children's Hospital which provides a large specialist community service for the city and a regional inpatient Tier 4 and Tertiary service. She is a mental health nurse by profession with over 27 years experience in both provider and commissioning organisations. Marie developed regional commissioning for CAMHS Tier 4 services in the West Midlands, which was the first in the country to commission services in this way, and in addition has a wealth of experience delivering mental health services in both rural and urban areas including as a Service Director across five London boroughs. Marie is passionate about patient experience and the involvement of user and carers within services. Through the nationally acclaimed evidence-based Meriden family intervention programme, she worked closely with users and carers to enhance services for families. She has been a member on several national project boards around mental health, including parental mental health, age appropriate services for under 18s, and CAMHS home treatment services. She has also presented at a range of international conferences.

Helen Hipkiss is Programme Consultant for Child Health, Child and Adult Safeguarding and is employed by NHS West Midlands. Helen has worked as a manager within the NHS for over 20 years within both commissioning and provider settings. She joined children's services as the CAMHS Strategic Manager for Walsall Primary Care Trust, before going on to be the CAMHS Regional Development Worker for Care Services Improvement Partnership (CSIP) and the National CAMHS Support Service (NCSS). Helen's current role is Programme Consultant covering 0–18 child health services. She is also responsible for child and adult safeguarding, as well as the delivery of the regional health visiting programme. Helen's areas of interest include CAMHS, children with disabilities, palliative care and safeguarding.

Tim McDougall is Nurse Consultant and Clinical Director for Tier 4 CAMHS and Trust-wide CAMHS at the Cheshire and Wirral NHS Foundation Trust. Tim has worked in a range of CAMHS settings including community child mental health teams, adolescent inpatient services and secure adolescent forensic services. With a national profile in CAMHS and with over 100 book and journal publications, Tim has spoken at national and European conferences about the mental health of children and adolescents. Tim was formerly Nurse Advisor for CAMHS at the Department of Health in England and was a member of the National Advisory Council for Children's Mental Health and Psychological Wellbeing. Tim is currently Chair of the UK Nurse Consultants in CAMHS Forum and the Quality Network for Inpatient CAMHS (QNIC) Executive Committee. He has been involved in the development of NICE guidelines on Psychosis and Schizophrenia in Children and Young People and Bipolar Disorder in Children, Young People and Adults.

Paul Mitchell is a Senior Mental Health Nurse currently working for Greater Manchester West NHS Foundation Trust as Clinical Lead for Mental Health Services in Hindley Young Offender Institution. Paul has worked in generic CAMHS but for most of his career has worked with adolescent offenders with mental health problems across the care pathway from Youth Offending Team work and community forensic assessments to adolescent forensic inpatient services. Paul has undertaken and published research on mental health screening, delivering interventions, and young people's attitudes to mental health services, and has presented at national and international conferences. Paul is currently working as Nurse Clinical Lead for the nationally commissioned Adolescent Forensic Service and is part of the NICE guideline development group for Conduct Disorders in Children and Young People.

Camilla Parker is a partner of Just Equality, a human rights and equality consultancy. She has worked as an independent consultant, specialising in mental health, disability and human rights law and policy since 1997, and has written, presented and trained extensively on issues relevant to these areas of law and policy, for specialist and non-specialist audiences, both nationally and internationally. Camilla is a member of the Law Society's Mental Health and Disability Committee. She was a member of an NHS Trust Board (non-executive Director, then Special Adviser) 2000–2006 and a Mental Health Act Commissioner 1995–2000. Camilla has a particular interest in the human rights of young people in need of mental health care, which is the subject of her part-time doctoral research at Cardiff Law School.

Angela Sergeant is a Nurse Consultant in Tier 4 CAMHS within Southern Health NHS Foundation Trust. Angela has worked in a range of CAMHS inpatient and community settings and she has been a key player in the commissioning of inpatient units. She also has expertise in the treatment of eating disorders in adolescents. She has a national profile in CAMHS, having conducted numerous reviews for the Health Advisory Service and Royal College of Psychiatrists, and External Consultancy Advisory Service throughout the UK. Angela has chaired and spoken at a number of national conferences regarding CAMHS issues and she has published and contributed to numerous books on CAMHS and eating disorders. Formerly a member of the Tier 4 Policy Implementation Group and NHS Confederation CAMHS sub group, Angela continues to represent nursing as a member of the Quality Network for Inpatient CAMHS (QNIC) advisory committee. She has also been a member of the development group for QNIC and Quality Network for Eating Disorders (QED) standards.

Cathy Street is an independent mental health researcher and consultant. Over the last ten years, she has held senior research, consultancy and management positions within a number of national mental health or young people's charities including YoungMinds, where she was Head of Research from 2000–2007, Youth Access, and most recently Rethink Mental Illness, where she was Young People's Research and Development Lead from 2009–2011. Cathy has led national evaluation and service improvement projects for various government departments and has published widely on children and young people's participation in mental health services; on services for young people from black and minority ethnic groups; on the provision and costs of Tier 4 and on new models of specialist CAMHS, including crisis and transition services.

Peter Thompson is a Senior Programme Manager at the Royal College of Psychiatrists. He has worked in the College Centre for Quality Improvement (CCQI) since 2004, working with accreditation and quality improvement projects. He manages the Quality Networks for Inpatient (QNIC) and Community (QNCC) CAMHS. Peter also manages the Quality Network for Perinatal Mental Health Services and oversees networks for forensic mental health services and therapeutic communities. He has developed service standards for a range of mental health services and has been a member of several national CAMHS steering groups including the CYP IAPT Service Transformation and Accreditation groups and the Tier 4 Policy Implementation Group. Peter has spoken about QNIC and QNCC at several national and international conferences.

Anne Worrall-Davies is Consultant Child and Adolescent Psychiatrist working across a CAMHS outreach and therapy service and an adolescent inpatient unit in Leeds Community Healthcare NHS Trust. She has a broad range of clinical experience, including paediatric liaison, outpatient CAMHS, and children's day services. Until 2008, Anne also worked as Senior Lecturer in Child and Adolescent Psychiatry at the University of Leeds with a research portfolio centring on evaluation of service models in lifespan mental health services. She retained a special interest in modernising Tier 4 services and has both written and researched in this area. Locally, Anne leads on NICE guidance implementation for CAMHS in Leeds, and nationally she has recently been part of the QNCC expert panel setting standards for intensive CAMHS.

ACKNOWLEDGEMENTS

The authors wish to thank the following people for their help and support in writing this book:

Dr Kirsty Smedley, Consultant Clinical Psychologist, Priory Group
Dr Justine Rothwell, Research Associate, SHIFT Trial
Dr Fiona Noble, Consultant Child and Adolescent Psychiatrist, Cheshire and Wirral Partnership NHS Foundation Trust.

FOREWORD

Lesley Hewson

As a young consultant in child and adolescent psychiatry, I remember the feeling of growing apprehension when assessing a young person at risk of suicide, or developing a psychosis. This was not about my inability to cope, nor insufficient training, but about the complete absence of services available to support the acute and complex needs of young people in crisis. In those days, CAMHS teams struggled on a daily basis to stem the flow of referrals, whilst managing the most worrying young people within only a very small Tier 2/3 community service. Out of area admissions were hard to arrange, and it felt as though we regularly juggled with risk, the only support being inappropriate stays in adult wards whilst we waited for a young person's bed to become available.

In 1998 we were inspired in Bradford to do something different. Adult services were successfully introducing a home-based approach into their service, and for us it no longer made sense that there was so little available locally for young people. Working closely with a forward thinking commissioner, and a creative CAMHS team, determined and willing to do things differently, we piloted a similar model of care. Home treatment, with individualised packages of care delivered by a seven-day service, underpinned by a young person and family centred approach, provided a flexible, alternative to inpatient care with an immediate effect on outcomes and improved user satisfaction.

This service has now been in place for 15 years, evaluated and further developed. Inpatient care has always remained an important component within this whole system of care. With appropriate and earlier interventions at home, enabling young people to remain engaged with friends, family and school, we found that they were often able to develop their own support mechanisms, promoting choice and empowerment and reducing the need for ongoing services.

Whilst the definition of Tier 4 has always included a wide range of highly specialist child and adolescent mental health services, too often the focus has been only on inpatient care, reflecting what was until relatively recently the prevailing approach in the management of the most troubled and complex young people. Developments in a range of evaluated, intensive and prescribed models of care have provided a considerable advance in our knowledge and understanding about service structure, content and style, including the early intervention programme, treatment foster care and multisystemic therapy.

This book quite rightly takes this broader approach to Tier 4 and in doing so provides an up-to-date account of the current state, including the evidence base, of those more specialised services, usually required by a comparative few, but that generally fall outside of mainstream, local community provision. Whilst the book outlines the many recent developments in the field, and in theory, we now know much more about the services that should be available to support young people with the most acute and complex mental health needs, everything is still far from perfect. Many services remain underfunded, and have developed without great attention to local need despite the aspiration of policymakers; no surprise then that many of the chapters end quite rightly by stressing that much more has still to be done.

The introduction of home treatment in Bradford was not without challenge and the importance of managers and clinicians working closely together cannot be overstated. Sadly in some services there is still protracted debate, at times almost irresolvable, between clinicians and their managers about the 'right way of providing services', delaying progress for young people. This is despite the key components of CAMHS services having been widely accepted since the National Service Framework (2004) and the ongoing development of NICE guidance. In my experience, those services that truly listen and respond to the views and opinions of the young people who use them, are more likely to avoid or find their way through these difficulties.

This book is published at a time of great uncertainty within the NHS. Changes in its core structure will have an effect on decision making and all aspects of how money will be spent in the future, including opening up the market to competition. For CAMHS to be most effective the services at each tier should be commissioned and provided as part of one complex yet integrated system: the quality of services at one level is inevitably dependent upon the quality of the services in the tier above and/or below. In addition, individualised care packages must be developed in partnership with the young person and their family or carers, and be flexible and responsive to their needs.

As Tier 4 commissioning becomes the responsibility of the NHS Commissioning Board one can only wait to see whether this approach will further improve the provision of a joined-up system of care or lead to further fragmentation. The Francis Report (2013) called for a culture where those using health services become 'the first and foremost consideration of the system and everyone who works in it'. It is crucial in the development of CAMHS that this principle is applied. The services described in this important book are aimed at the most troubled, and at times troublesome, young people in our communities. This book should ensure that the progress made in delivering services to this group continues. It is in everyone's interest that this book is widely read.

Dr Lesley Hewson OBE was Vice-chair of the National Advisory Council for Children's Mental Health and Psychological Wellbeing (2008–2011), an independent Ministerial Advisory Group established to hold the government to account in delivering the recommendations of the National CAMHS Review (1988). She was formerly Clinical Director of Bradford CAMHS and Consultant in Child and Adolescent Psychiatry in Bradford from 1988 until 2009 where she pioneered the development of home treatment. She now works independently.

ABBREVIATIONS AND ACRONYMS

AACAP	American Academy of Child and Adolescent Psychiatry
ADHD	attention deficit hyperactivity disorder
ADTP	adolescent day treatment program
AIMS	Accreditation in Adult Mental Health Services
AMBIT	adolescent mentalisation based integrative therapy
AMHP	approved mental health professional
AMHS	adult mental health services
AOT	assessment and outreach team
ASC	autism spectrum conditions
A-SPS	Adapted SAD Persons Scale
BHTS	Bradford Home Treatment Service
BNF	British National Formulary
BNFC	British National Formulary for Children
CA	Children Act
CAMHS	child and adolescent mental health services
CAMHSSS	CAMHS Service Satisfaction Scale
CAPA	choice and partnership approach
CAPE	Care Placements Evaluation
CASSP	Federal National Institute of Mental Health Child and Adolescent Service System Program
CBT	cognitive behavioural therapy
CCG	clinical commissioning group
CCQI	Royal College of Psychiatrists Centre for Quality Improvment
CFWI	Centre for Workforce Intelligence
CGAS	Children's Global Assessment Scale
CHAT	Comprehensive Health Assessment Tool
CHIMAT	Child and Maternal Health Observatory

CHRT	crisis resolution home treatment team
CIN	Child in Need
CIP	cost improvement programme
CIRS	CAMHS Inpatient Referral Study
CITT	community intensive therapy team
CORC	CAMHS Outcome Research Consortium
CPA	Care Programme Approach
CPD	Continuing Professional Development
CPN	community psychiatric nurse
CQUIN	Commissioning for Quality and Innovation
CT	computed tomography
CWDC	Children's Workforce Development Council
DBT	dialectical behaviour therapy
DCSF	Department for Children, Schools and Families
DfE	Department for Education
DUP	duration of untreated psychosis
EARL	Early Assessment Risk List
ECG	electrocardiogram
EDDP	eating disorders day programme
EEG	electroencephalography
EIP	Early Intervention in Psychosis
EPSE	extra pyramidal side effects
ERASOR	Estimate of Risk of Adolescent Sexual Offense Recidivism
FAD	Family Assessment Device
FFT	functional family therapy
GBO	goal-based outcomes
GP	general practitioner
HAS	Health Advisory Service
HASCAS	Health and Social Care Advisory Service
HBTS	home-based therapy service
HEE	Health Education England
HoNOSCA	Health of the Nation Outcomes Scale (Child and Adolescent Mental Health)
HWB	Health and Wellbeing Board
ICD	International Classification of Diseases
ICM	intensive case management
ICOS	intensive community outreach service
IICAPS	Intensive In-Home Child and Adolescent Psychiatric Service
IQ	intelligence quotient
ISSP	Intensive Supervision and Surveillance Programme
J-SOAP	Juvenile Sex Offender Assessment Protocol
KEEP	Keeping Foster and Kinship Parents Supported and Trained
LAC	looked after children
LAT	local area team

LETB	local education and training boards
MACI	Millon Adolescent Clinical Inventory
MCA	Mental Capacity Act
MDFT	multidimensional family therapy
MDT	multi disciplinary team
MHA	Mental Health Act
MRI	magnetic resonance imaging
MST	multisystemic therapy
MST-CAN	multisystemic therapy for child abuse and neglect
MST-PSB	multisystemic therapy for problem sexual behaviour
MST-SA	multisystemic therapy for substance misuse
MTFC	multidimensional treatment foster care
MTFC-A	multidimensional treatment foster care (adolescents)
MTFC-C	multidimensional treatment foster care (children)
MTFC-P	multidimensional treatment foster care (prevention)
NAC	National Advisory Council
NCB	National Commissioning Board
NCSS	National CAMHS Support Service
NHS	National Health Service
NICE	National Institute for Care Excellence
NIHR	National Institute for Health Research
NIMHE	National Institute for Mental Health in England
NREPP	National Registry of Evidence-based Programs and Practices
NSF	National Service Framework
NWW	new ways of working
NYAS	National Youth Advocacy Service
OCD	obsessive compulsive disorder
OLSC	Oregon Social Learning Center
ONS	Office for National Statistics
PCL-YV	Psychopathy Checklist - Youth Version
PCT	primary care trust
PPI	patient and public involvement
PSHE	personal, social and health education
PTSD	post-traumatic stress disorder
QIPP	quality, innovation, productivity and prevention
QNCC	Quality Network for Community CAMHS
QNIC	Quality Network for Inpatient Child and Adolescent Mental Health Services
QNIC ROM	Quality Network for Inpatient Child and Adolescent Mental Health Services Routine Outcome Measurement Service
QOF	Quality and Outcomes Framework
RCT	randomised controlled trial
RTC	residential treatment center
RC	responsible clinician

RCP	Royal College of Psychiatrists
RCPCH	Royal College of Paediatrics and Child Health
SAMHSA	Substance Abuse and Mental Health Services Administration
SAVRY	structured assessment of violence risk in youth
SCID	Structured Clinical Interview for DSM-IV Axis II Personality Disorders
SCIE	Social Care Institute for Excellence
SCT	supervised community treatment
SDQ	Strengths and Difficulties Questionnaire
SEN	special educational need
SHIFT	self harm intervention family therapy
SIFA	Screening Interview for Adolescents
SNASA	Salford Needs Assessment for Adolescents
SPC	summary of product characteristics
SSRI	selective serotonin reuptake inhibitor
START	Systemic Therapy for At Risk Teens
STEPS-B	Services for Teens Engaging in Problem Sexual Behaviour
TAC	team around the child
TAF	team around the family
WHO	World Health Organisation
YJB	Youth Justice Board
YOS	Youth Offending Service
YOT	Youth Offending Team
ZPC	zone of parental control

INTRODUCTION

Tim McDougall and Andy Cotgrove

The need to develop a comprehensive range of services for young people requiring highly specialised mental healthcare and treatment has been a UK policy objective since the early 1990s. It is nearly a decade since the National Service Framework (NSF) for Children, Young People and Maternity Services stated that young people must be able to access Tier 4 child and adolescent mental health services (CAMHS). The NSF defined these as intensive outpatient services; assertive outreach teams; inpatient residential and secure provision; or other highly specialised assessment, consultation and intervention services (Department of Health 2004). A decade on and despite clear policy declarations, highly specialised mental health services for children and young people have been neglected in many areas of the UK and in some areas have not developed at all.

The impact of this is only partly apparent. Gaps in access to hospital, intensive community and home-based services for children and young people have historically led to care and treatment in inappropriate settings such as paediatric or adult mental health wards (Worrall et al. 2004; McDougall & Bodley-Scott 2008). In some cases, young people have been unable to access services at all. They have been either too young or too old, or too ill or not ill enough. In addition, some young people end up in the health system, and in particular admitted to hospital, because of unmet social care needs. The longer-term costs of untreated mental health problems, through lack of access to appropriate treatments and psychosocial interventions, may take years to manifest. Most mental health problems start before the age of 25. Half of all lifetime mental disorders begin by age 14 and three-quarters start before a young person reaches their mid-20s (Kim-Cohen et al. 2003; Maughan & Kim-Cohen 2005). The King's Fund has projected that the annual cost of mental healthcare will increase from what was £22.5 billion in 2007 to at least £32.6 billion by 2026 (Crone et al. 2008).

The case for early intervention is unequivocal. Treatment at an earlier stage is likely to be more effective and less costly than that which will be needed over a lifetime if the opportunity for prevention and early intervention is missed (Knapp & Parsonage 2001; Royal College of Psychiatrists 2010). In 2011 an independent report for the UK Government highlighted a range of intensive community services that are known to be both clinically effective and cost effective for vulnerable children and their families. These included multisystemic therapy (MST), functional family therapy (FFT) and multidimensional treatment foster care (MTFC) (HM Government 2011). It is not only mental disorder that intensive community and home-based services can address effectively. There is a strong case for developing and testing interventions for several groups of vulnerable children and young people, such as children placed for adoption and adopted children at risk of placement breakdown and their families (Department for Education 2011). For example, multiple evaluations have shown that FFT, provided with treatment fidelity, reduces criminal recidivism, out of home placements or referral of other adolescents in the family for extra help from children's services by between 25 per cent and 55 per cent (Alexander et al. 1998).

At the time of writing this book the National Health Service (NHS) and children's sector is going through large-scale, unprecedented change. Public services are expected to make huge efficiency savings. In some areas we are starting to see the impact of disinvestment in front-line services. Child and adolescent mental health services are becoming dangerously overstretched and there has been a steady increase in referrals, greater complexity of need in the people specialist services are seeing, and higher expectations from multi-agency partners. This is in the context of a dilution of staff skills as part of cost improvement programmes, longer waiting lists and a shrinking workforce of professionals trained and experienced in evidence-based treatment interventions. On the other hand, we have an ever expanding evidence base on which to draw. Services can be targeted where we know they will be most effective, and interventions that are proving to be ineffective can be stopped.

Chapter 1 explores what we mean by highly specialised mental health services. We refer to what are commonly described as tertiary Tier 4 services, and in Chapter 2 discuss how these fit with the wider tiered model of care and in particular local community Tier 3 services. However, the tiered model has not been without criticism – particularly from local authority critics, many of whom prefer the nomenclature of universal, targeted and specialist services.

For many years the terms inpatient units and Tier 4 provision have been thought of as synonymous. This is misleading, unhelpful and may have partly contributed to an historic neglect of Tier 4 commissioning (McDougall et al. 2008). Chapter 3 discusses the role of inpatient beds as part of a wider system of interventions, the component parts of which are rarely available as comprehensive services. It is important to say, however, that the majority of young people with severe, complex or persistent mental health problems never require hospital admission. Instead they are treated in primary services or by community-based specialist teams, some of which we describe later in the book.

Chapter 4 explores day services. According to the Quality Network for Inpatient Child and Adolescent Mental Health Services (QNIC), about half of UK day services are linked to inpatient units and the majority of inpatient units have a day programme. It is very difficult to classify day services due to the enormous range in milieu and interventions they provide. However, day services commonly offer support and transition to community services following inpatient admission through intensive five day-per-week treatment packages. Some offer specialist programmes for younger children with developmental disorders such as autism or neuro-psychiatric disorders, and intensive intervention aimed at improving family functioning in situations of family breakdown.

Early intervention services for children and young people with psychosis are described in Chapter 5. This is followed by a chapter on treatment foster care which is aimed at children and young people who may be on developmental trajectories towards crime and antisocial behaviour. Standard 9 of the National Service Framework for Children, Young People and maternity Services (Department of Health 2004) suggests that in order to meet the mental health needs of children and young people with severe, challenging and complex problems a network of care is required which includes therapeutic fostering services.

Psychological treatment is unlikely to be successful without a stable care arrangement. Due to the difficulty in achieving such stability, there is a recognised need to provide professional support and training for foster carers. Chapter 6 discusses treatment foster care where parents are 'trained' by programme supervisors in skills of effective supervision, limit setting and reinforcement. Although it is relatively expensive to provide, treatment foster care has been shown to have positive outcomes in terms of reducing behaviour problems, lowering placement disruption rates and improving foster parent retention (Chamberlain & Reid 1998).

Chapter 7 focuses on MST. Like treatment foster care this is a US developed treatment and intervention programme which has been piloted in the UK. MST is an intensive, manualised family-based approach which has been used successfully with young people with conduct disorder, antisocial behaviour and substance misuse (Henggeler et al. 1999). It has been shown to reduce out of home placements, and has been linked to reducing rates of reoffending and improved family functioning. Whilst MST is resource intensive and again is relatively expensive to provide, evidence from the US and UK suggests that it may be effective in optimising outcomes for young people and reducing the future burden on the public sector, particularly the criminal justice system.

The National Commissioning Board has specified that home treatment teams should be commissioned as part of the integrated range of Tier 4 services (Department of Health 2012). Reviews of home treatment studies have found that they can be helpful for young people with a range of mental health problems including acute psychosis, eating disorders and suicidal behaviour, and seem to largely avert admission to inpatient services without a significant deterioration in mental health and social functioning (Worrall-Davies & Kiernan 2005). Patient and relative satisfaction has been evaluated as part of adult studies, and has been found to be higher in home care compared with hospital admission (Kurtz 2009). Home-based treatment and therapy services for children and young people are discussed in Chapter 8 and both community and secure forensic interventions are described in Chapter 9.

The Royal College of Psychiatrists (2006) suggests that the views of children, young people and their carers should actively be sought by clinicians, managers and commissioners and incorporated into strategies for Tier 4 CAMHS service delivery. It is vital that children, young people and parents are involved in every aspect of service planning, delivery and evaluation, and what they tell us about the services we commission and provide are discussed in Chapter 10. Chapter 11 highlights the importance of planning transition for children and young people requiring hospital, intensive community and home-based services.

For many years Tier 4 commissioning across the UK has been subject to wide geographical variation. Progress in commissioning which is strategic and needs led has been extremely slow, and commissioning for the development of community-based alternatives to inpatient beds have not come to fruition in many areas of the country. As this book was being written responsibility for the commissioning of what will broadly be known as Tier 4 CAMHS was transitioning from regional specialised commissioning groups to NHS England. Chapter 12 addresses the commissioning of Tier 4 CAMHS and other intensive community and home-based services.

It is important that services are high quality and based on the best available evidence. Chapter 13 describes a range of quality standards that underpin the commissioning and provision of hospital, intensive community and home-based services. The legal framework surrounding the care and treatment of young people requiring hospital, intensive community and home-based services is complex. Therefore Chapter 14 covers the key aspects of the Children Act, Mental Health Act and Mental Capacity Act and the interrelationship between these legislative frameworks as they are applied to children and young people with mental disorder. It is essential that the workforce required to provide hospital, intensive community and home-based services for children and young people are competent, capable and supported. The final chapter discusses workforce planning, training and staff development.

In summary, the role, commissioning and management of Tier 4 CAMHS are often poorly understood. Commissioners, organisations providing Tier 4 CAMHS and professionals providing day to day services require high quality information resources to inform their practice. Together with the chapter authors who are experts in their subject areas, we combine our collective clinical, research and service improvement experience together in this book. It is by no means a comprehensive account of inpatient, intensive community and home-based services. However, we hope the book will go some way in assisting all who are responsible for supporting children and young people with mental health problems, whether they are parents, clinicians, managers, commissioners or policymakers. Together, we have a real opportunity to make a difference.

References

Alexander, J., Barton, C., Gordon, D., Grotpeter, J., Hansson, K., Harrison, R., Mears, S., Mihalic, S., Parsons, B., Pugh, C., Schulman, S., Waldron, H. & Sexton, T. (1998). Functional Family Therapy: Blueprints for Violence Prevention. In: Elliot, D. (Ed.) *Blueprints for Violence Prevention*. Boilder, CO: Center for the Study and Prevention of Violence, Institute of Behavioral Science, University of Colorado.

Chamberlain, P. & Reid, J. B. (1998). Comparison of two community alternatives to incarceration for chronic juvenile offenders. *Journal of Consulting and Clinical Psychology*, 66, 624–633.

Crone. P., Dhanasiri, S., Patel, A., Knapp, M. & Lawton-Smith, S. (2008). *Paying the Price: the cost of mental health care in England to 2026*. London: King's Fund.

Department for Education. (2011). *Prospectus: delivering intensive interventions for looked after children and those on the edge of custody and their families*. London: HMSO.

Department of Health. (2012). *Clinical Advisory Group for Prescribed Services: final recommendations*. London: HMSO.

Department of Health. (2012). *Clinical Advisory Group for Prescribed Services: final recommendations*. London: HMSO.

Department of Health. (2004). *National Service Framework for Children, Young People and Maternity Services: standard 9: the mental health and psychological well-being of children and young people*. London: HMSO.

Henggeler, S. W., Rowland, M. D., Randall, J., Ward, D. M., Pickrel, S. G., Cunningham, P. B., Miller, S., Edwards, J., Zealberg, J. J., Hand, L. E. & Santos, A. B. (1999) Home-based multisystemic therapy as an alternative to the hospitalisation of youths in psychiatric crisis: clinical outcomes. *Journal of American Academy of Child and Adolescent Psychiatry*, 38(11), 1331–1339.

HM Government. (2011). *Early Intervention: the next steps*. London: HMSO.

Kim-Cohen, J., Caspi, A., Moffitt, T., Harrington, H. et al. (2003). Prior juvenile diagnoses in adults with mental disorder: developmental follow back of a prospective longitudinal cohort. *Archives of General Psychiatry*, 60(7), 709–717.

Knapp, M. & Parsonage, M. (2001). *Mental Health Promotion and Mental Illness Prevention: the economic case*. London: HMSO.

Kurtz, Z. (2009). *The Evidence Base to Guide Development of Tier 4 CAMHS*. London: HMSO.

McDougall, T. & Bodley-Scott, S. (2008). Too much too young: under 18s on adult mental health wards. *Mental Health Practice*, 11(6), 12–15.

McDougall, T., Worrall-Davies, A., Hewson, L., Richardson, G. & Cotgrove, A. (2008). Tier 4 Child and Adolescent Mental Health Services: inpatient care, day services and alternatives: an overview of Tier 4 CAMHS provision in the UK. *Child and Adolescent Mental Health*, 13(4), 173–180.

Maughan, B. & Kim-Cohen, J. (2005). Continuities between childhood and adult life. *British Journal of Psychiatry*, 187, 301–303.

Royal College of Psychiatrists. (2010). *No Health without Public Mental Health: the case for action*. London: RCP.

Royal College of Psychiatrists. (2006). *Building and Sustaining Specialist Child and Adolescent Mental Health Services*. London: RCP.

Worrall-Davies, A. & Kiernan, K. (2005). *Using a Virtual Team: an evaluation of the Bradford CAMHS intensive home treatment approach*. Leeds: Bradford Children and Young People's Partnership, University of Leeds.

Worrall, A., O'Herlihey, A., Banerjee, S., Jaffa, T., Lelliot, P., Hill, P., Scott, A. & Brook, H. (2004). Inappropriate admission of young people with mental disorder to adult psychiatric wards and paediatric wards: cross sectional study of 6 months activity. *British Medical Journal*, doi: 10.1136/bmj.38058.605787.AE.

1

WHAT DO WE MEAN BY SPECIALIST HOSPITAL, INTENSIVE COMMUNITY AND HOME-BASED SERVICES?

Tim McDougall

Key points

- One of the most important landmarks in the history of CAMHS strategy in the UK was the 1995 NHS Health Advisory Service's 'tiered model' of service delivery. Nearly 20 years since its inception the tiered model remains the preferred framework to organise the commissioning, management and delivery of mental health services for children and young people with mental health problems and disorders in the UK.
- The evidence base for Tier 4 CAMHS is in its infancy. Evidence for some services is poorly developed, and for others it is based on US or European services where systems for commissioning and providing healthcare are different to those in the UK.
- The predominant model of intervention in Tier 4 CAMHS for young people in the UK remains admission to hospital. The models of care that exist as alternatives to admission are intensive community and day care, intensive outpatient treatment and home-based services. However, these are not routinely available across the UK and in some areas are few and far between or not available at all.
- The effectiveness of hospital, intensive community and home-based services depends on a number of essential factors. These include early intervention, a thorough knowledge of the child or young person, interventions that focus on difficulties and problems across multiple domains of functioning, adherence to treatment and completion of the therapeutic programme.
- The delivery of effective interventions for children requiring hospital, intensive community and home-based services depends crucially on an appropriately trained, skilled and experienced workforce. Working with children and young people with complex psychosocial needs can be a challenging and emotionally draining process. It is therefore important that those providing care and treatment interventions have access to supervision and support from skilled practitioners

Introduction

This chapter discusses what we mean by hospital, intensive community and home-based services in the UK policy and planning context. Definitions offered by clinicians and commissioners are compared. The evidence base for the range of services that are broadly referred to as Tier 4 is summarised, and good practice distilled from what is known about the success of existing services is discussed.

Background

The most important strategic document to set the context in which CAMHS in the UK have evolved was the NHS Health Advisory Service (HAS) report, *Together we Stand* (NHS Health Advisory Service 1995). This provided a detailed summary of the characteristics of nationwide CAMHS, with chapters on epidemiology, needs assessment, service principles, and the commissioning and provision of services. The report led to widespread use of the acronym 'CAMHS' and applied the four tiered framework to help promote the important message that child and adolescent mental health is everyone's business. In this report Tier 4 CAMHS were described as follows:

> Tier 4 provides for highly specific and complex problems which require considerable resources. These include, for example, inpatient psychiatric provision for adolescents, secure provision, specialist facilities for those with sensory handicaps, very specialised services (outpatient and inpatient) for young people with severe eating disorders, specialised neuropsychiatric out-day and inpatient services and consultation services for rare paediatric disorders.
>
> (NHS Health Advisory Service 1995)

Whilst it has not been without criticism the 'tiered model' of service delivery remains the preferred framework to organise the commissioning, management and delivery of mental health services for children and young people with mental health problems and disorders in the UK. The ways in which the tiered model operates, both by design and by accident, are discussed further in Chapter 2 which focuses on the clinical pathways to hospital, intensive community and home-based services. However, for the purpose of setting the context for this chapter and the book which follows, it is outlined in Figure 1.1.

Tier 1

Parents and professionals in primary, universal or front-line services are usually the first to recognise that children and young people may be struggling. These include general practitioners (GPs), teachers, school nurses and health visitors. Tier 1 services are those in which children and young people receive day-to-day healthcare or education. They are provided in GP practices, schools and social care settings, and workers in these settings should have a basic understanding about self-harm and know how to refer a child for primary care or more specialist assessment.

Tier 1
Services at primary level by professionals providing non-specialist CAMHS in health, education, social services and youth justice settings. This involves mental health promotion, early identification of mental health problems and in some cases, treatment for less severe mental health problems e.g. sleep, temper tantrums, behaviour problems at home/school and bereavement.

Professionals
Health visitors, Portage Practice nurses, School nurses, Sure Start worker, GPs
Voluntary sector workers, Youth workers, Teachers, Healthy Schools Project Workers
Social workers, Family support workers.

Tier 2
Individual professionals working relatively independently from other services, but relating to each other through a network. They provide training and consultation to Tier 1 workers, outreach to identify complex, severe or persistent mental disorders and sign-post children and young people to specialist CAMHS at Tiers 2 or 3.

Professionals
Clinical psychologist, Educational psychologist
Child and adolescent psychiatrist, YOT health nurse specialist, Primary mental health worker
Community paediatrician, Hospital paediatrician.

Most children with mental health problems will be seen at Tiers 1 and 2

Tier 3
Specialist multi-disciplinary child and adolescent teams

Professionals
Psychiatrists, mental health nurses, psychologists, social workers, family therapists and others providing assessment and treatment for children and young people with complex, persistent or severe mental disorders. Assessment for referrals to Tier 4.
Provision of support and training for Tier 2 and offer consultation to Tier 1 professionals.

Tier 4
Specialist multi-disciplinary child and adolescent teams.
In-patient child and adolescent units may also have support from occupational therapists, speech and language therapists and creative therapists who specialise in art, music, drama or play therapy.

| In-patient child and adolescent units Day services | Intensive home based treatment teams / crisis outreach services | Out-patient services for eating disorders; neuropsychiatric problems; sexual abuse; OCD, etc. |

FIGURE 1.1   NHS Health Advisory tiered model of service delivery (1995) (Source: McDougall, 2006)

Tier 2

Tier 2 services are provided by professionals with additional training or expertise in child and adolescent mental health. Their role is to provide direct assessment or treatment for individual children and young people with less complex problems than those requiring most specialist interventions at Tier 3 or 4 services. They also provide support, guidance and training for Tier 1 professionals providing front-line services.

Tier 3

Professionals working in services at Tiers 1 and 2 must be able to access specialist CAMHS where they have concerns about the mental health of a child or young person they are working with. Tier 3 services are dedicated multidisciplinary teams providing comprehensive assessment, treatment and consultation services for children and young people with complex, persistent or severe mental health needs and disorders. Tier 3 teams usually comprise psychiatrists, psychologists, nurses, family therapists, social workers and other therapists. They offer a range of psychological and pharmacological treatments.

Tier 4

Tier 4 services are highly specialised tertiary CAMHS and include inpatient child and adolescent units, specialised eating disorders services and forensic CAMHS, as well as multi-agency services such as home treatment services, community support teams and crisis teams. It is these services which are described in detail throughout this book. The Royal College of Psychiatrists (2006) also refer to 'non NHS Tier 4 settings' including specialist residential schools and social care homes, specialist foster care, enhanced social services residential placements and local authority secure units. The College suggests that such settings may or may not have mental health as a focus of their work and may or may not have specialist mental health workers in their teams.

Policy definitions

A significant landmark in the development of Tier 4 services was the National Service Framework (NSF) for Children, Young People and Maternity Services (Department of Health 2004). In this framework for commissioning and providing children's services, Tier 4 CAMHS were defined as follows:

> Highly specialised comprising intensive outpatient services; assertive outreach teams; inpatient residential and secure provision; and other highly specialised assessment, consultation and intervention services. Amongst the highly specialist services, inpatient psychiatric units for both children and adolescents, but separately provided to ensure that the developmental needs of different age ranges are met, are essential resources, representing 'the intensive care of child mental health'. A network of care is required in each locality for children and young people with severe, challenging

and complex problems. This will promote collaborative working between services such as therapeutic fostering, pupil referral units, secure units, adolescent in-patient units and children's homes. Tier 3 and Tier 4 have a role in providing mental health services to secure units (e.g. secure children's homes, secure training centres and young offenders institutions), residential education and residential care, together with other intensive community settings, e.g. specialist fostering.

To achieve this vision for Tier 4 services the Department of Health made a number of policy declarations and set standards for service providers and commissioners. Multi-agency and specialist commissioning and planning were to drive and shape Tier 4 services according to need and best practice, enabling the delivery of a volume of services that would encompass the challenges of demand, capacity, diversity and capability. Emergency care, general and specialist inpatient services (e.g. eating disorders, forensic, medium secure and learning disability) would be available for children and young people from each locality. The numbers of beds was to be matched to need for each locality. Patients who should be admitted on clinical grounds would not be refused access due to limitation of resources such as bed availability.

Primary Care Trusts (PCTs) and local authorities were to ensure that a network of care was developed in partnership for the provision of Tier 4 services, and that written criteria for admission were to be available and understood by professionals working with children and young people. Health providers of Tier 4 CAMHS were expected work in collaboration with specialist education, social care and youth justice provision to provide a network of services for children and young people with severe, challenging and complex problems. Furthermore, PCTs and local authorities were to ensure that local networks of care were developed between Tier 3 and Tier 4 services to include assertive outreach and day care as well as inpatient and community services. Specialist CAMHS were to become involved in the provision of mental health services to secure units, residential education and residential care, together with other intensive community settings such as within specialist fostering. There was to be close collaboration and liaison with adult mental health services.

The NSF stated that there needed to be a shared understanding of the level of care required on discharge from inpatient services and the appropriate resources available across community services. Shared aftercare arrangements and transition protocols between CAMHS and general adult psychiatric services were to be agreed and subject to audit. When children and young people were unavoidably placed on paediatric or adult psychiatric wards, there was to be collaboration and joint working between child health, adult mental health and CAMHS professionals.

To help map progress against standard 9 of the NSF the University of Durham led a CAMHS mapping project which gave more detail to an expanded definition of 'Tier 4 Special Care Teams'. Special care included the provision of treatment or care more often than weekly or twice weekly through inpatient care, outreach support and intensive aftercare. Day services and intensive fostering also fell into this category, as did intensive home visiting and/or frequent and unscheduled attendance at day care to avert the need for residential care.

The new 'post-NSF' world

Nearly a decade on, the NSF may soon be replaced by a new strategy, and it is disappointing that the range of services and the underpinning standards that were in the framework have still not been developed in some parts of the UK.

Nearly two decades following the introduction of the tiered model in CAMHS, responsibility for commissioning Tier 4 services across England has transferred from local clinical commissioning groups to NHS England. The clinical reference group that has been advising the Department of Health on what Tier 4 services should comprise have developed the specifications that will inform commissioning, and ultimately service provision.

The new specification which will drive commissioning and service provision defines Tier 4 CAMHS as follows:

> Tier 4 Child and Adolescent Mental Health services will include in-patients and bespoke packages of care for intensive day care services (as an alternative to admission) provided by Specialist Child and Adolescent Mental Health Centres. In addition, this will include associated non-admitted care including out-reach when delivered as part of a provider network.
>
> (Department of Health 2012)

It is positive that this process has been influenced by clinicians who know and understand the realities of working in hospital, intensive community and home-based services. It remains to be seen whether the new commissioning arrangements under the responsibility and leadership of NHS England will lead to better access for children and young people to hospital, intensive community and home-based services.

Clinical definitions

In defining specialist CAMHS Ann York and colleagues define Tier 4 provision as very specialised services in residential, day patient or outpatient settings for young people with severe and/or complex problems requiring a combination or intensity of interventions that cannot be provided by Tier 3 (York & Lamb 2005).

Similarly, Kurtz (2009) comments that until recently the idea of Tier 4 specialist CAMHS was synonymous with psychiatric inpatient provision, sometimes with day hospitals attached. She goes on to suggest that Tier 4 has more recently come to be understood as multifaceted with multi-agency services that can include in-reach, outreach, intensive and crisis community initiatives, day provision, therapeutic fostering and other services that may be described as 'wraparound'. Kurtz goes on to predict that the development of intensive community teams is likely to alter the focus of inpatient treatment, with increasing emphasis on symptom stabilisation and minimum necessary change before rapid discharge of the child or young person.

However, Tier 4 services are also sometimes defined by their exclusions. The Royal College of Psychiatrists (2006) points out that many Tier 4 CAMHS exclude young people whose behavioural problems are driven by learning disability, conduct disorder or substance misuse. Recognising this as representing significant service gaps the College suggests that young people with these problems must be taken into account in planning Tier 4 services.

The evidence base for Tier 4 CAMHS

Despite growing concern about the prevalence of mental health problems in children and young people the evidence base is in its infancy and does little to guide the development of services (National Institute for Health Research 2008). Evidence for some services is patchy, and for others the evidence claim is based on US services where systems for commissioning and providing healthcare are fragmented by multiple health insurers and providers (Burns et al. 1995). Historically, the commissioning of Tier 4 services has been driven more by local interest than strategic planning, and has been lacking in good quality information about need and demand (McDougall et al. 2008).

In many areas of health research, the populations of people studied have similar disorders, similar symptom profiles and developmental level and similar socio-economic status. This is not so in research focusing on highly specialised mental health treatments and intervention services. Patient populations are heterogeneous, the numbers of people who are studied are relatively small, and the culture and philosophy of intervention varies from service to service, from team to team and from individual to individual. Outcomes are sometimes investigated using a number of different scales. This makes robust comparison and multi-centre studies of large scale treatments very difficult to carry out in what are essentially heterogeneous Tier 4 CAMHS.

Despite the common adoption of the Declaration of Helsinki there is substantial variation between European countries in the requirements for approval by a research ethics committee (Meenaghan et al. 2007). The UK Department of Health guidelines in relation to research ethics and governance present significant challenges to undertaking mental health service research within the National Health Service (NHS). This is partly due to a high profile inquiry into a children's hospital in the 1990s where researchers had retained children's organs without parental consent (House of Commons 2001).

Drawing on the experience of gaining ethical approval for a study on young people referred but not admitted to Tier 4 units, Meenaghan and colleagues (2007) report how ethical research and governance procedures can get in the way of conducting health service research. They suggest that the level of bureaucracy involved may threaten the quality of policy development and service planning. Scandinavian countries have had more success in carrying out large-scale longitudinal outcome research on children with psychiatric disorders. This is partly due to less arduous research requirements (Hearnshaw 2004) and partly because of access to national healthcare registers (Thomsen 1996; Sourander & Turunen 1999).

Alternatives to inpatient care for children and young people

Since the tiered model of service provision became operational, it is unfortunate that the terms Tier 4 CAMHS and inpatient beds have been used interchangeably. In recent years, alternatives to inpatient care for children and young people have been developed and described in policy, research summaries and systematic reviews (Department of Health 2004; National Institute for Health Research 2008).

Many countries place emphasis on providing mental health services in the least restrictive setting, recognising that some children and young people may need to be admitted to hospital. As a result there are a range of mental health services to manage young people with serious mental health problems in community or outpatient settings who are at risk of being admitted to hospital. Lamb (2009) reviewed the evidence for alternatives to hospital admission for children and adolescents with severe and complex mental health problems. Although various adult studies compared hospital with intensive case management and assertive outreach, she could find little high quality research into the effectiveness of interventions with children and young people. This of course does not mean that such services are not effective, rather that there is a need for more high quality research.

Evidence has shown the need to reconfigure traditional provision for young people requiring Tier 4 CAMHS to ensure services are multifaceted and multi-organisational, offering a combination of in-reach, outreach, intensive and crisis community provision, day care, intensive fostering and other services that may be described as 'wraparound'. McDougall and colleagues (2008) point to the need for a 'mixed economy' of inpatient provision and complementary home-based and community outreach services.

Similarly, the Royal College of Psychiatrists propose that intensive community treatment programmes should be developed in the context of, and closely linked with, well resourced Tier 3 services and accessible age appropriate Tier 4 inpatient facilities. The College suggests that such provision should include day units; crisis teams, intensive community support teams, outreach teams, home treatment teams; enhanced paediatric wards, specialist adolescent wards; and liaison community mental health teams for 16- to 18-year-olds (Royal College of Psychiatrists 2006).

Hospital admission versus community alternatives

Several studies have compared hospital admission with intensive community or home-based alternatives (Woolston 1998; Mattejat et al. 2001). There were few differences in relation to clinical outcomes or broader outcomes such as how children coped at home or in school. No randomised evidence has been identified comparing intensive day treatment, intensive case management, residential care or therapeutic foster care with inpatient care or another alternative type of care (National Institute for Health Research 2009).

A randomised controlled trial (RCT) by Gowers and colleagues compared inpatient, specialist outpatient and Tier 3 CAMHS treatment for young people with an eating disorder. Their study indicated that whilst young people make considerable progress in all services, neither inpatient nor specialist outpatient services demonstrated advantages over general CAMHS treatment (Gowers et al. 2007).

However, some treatment outcomes associated with some models of intensive community-based care are similar to those following treatment in hospital and may be sustained longer after follow-up (Green & Worrall-Davies 2008). Schwartz and Wernert

(1993) showed that community-based treatments reduced admission rates and length of stay for severely mentally ill adolescents in a US sample. Such alternative services are cheaper than inpatient care and support the principle of 'least restriction', a concept enshrined in mental health and human rights legislation as well as NHS England's specification for Tier 4 CAMHS (Department of Health 2012).

Despite these underpinning principles, alternatives to inpatient services for young people have not generally been commissioned and provided in the UK (Shetty 2007). Whilst the *National CAMHS Review* (Department for Children, Schools and Families 2008) suggested that more Tier 4 services were providing alternatives to inpatient care on an intensive outreach basis, in some areas of the UK what have been described as *alternatives* to inpatient care have been misunderstood as a *replacement for* inpatient care. Consequently, the predominant model of service provision for young people across the UK has remained one of hospital admission.

A systematic review as part of mapping of alternatives to inpatient provision across urban and rural areas of the UK showed that the available but limited models of care were early intervention in psychosis (EIP) services, intensive day care, intensive outpatient treatment, and home-based services (National Institute for Health Research 2009) (see Box 1.1).

However, the National Institute for Health Research (NIHR) list is not exhaustive, and several other service models exist in the US, Europe and the UK. These include functional family therapy, multi-family therapy and case management as well as what might broadly be termed 'wraparound' services. Some of these services are mentioned in Chapter 8.

Similarly, in her review of Tier 4 CAMHS in England, Kurtz (2007) highlighted a number of promising initiatives to develop a range of services to help prevent inappropriate hospital admission. These include assertive outreach and home treatment teams, EIP services and specialist outpatient services such as dialectical behaviour therapy (DBT).

BOX 1.1 Alternatives to inpatient care

- Multi systemic therapy (Henggeler et al. 1999; Littell et al. 2005; Rowland et al. 2005)
- Day hospital (Grizenko et al. 1993a, 1993b)
- Case management
- Intensive specialist outpatient service (Gowers et al. 2007; Byford et al. 2007)
- Home treatment (Winsberg et al. 1980; Mattejat et al. 2001; Schmidt et al. 2006)
- Family preservation services (Pecora et al. 1991; Wilmshurst 2002; Evans et al. 2003)
- Therapeutic foster care
- Services in residential care
- Home treatment
- Intensive outreach
- Crisis intervention
- Early intervention for psychosis

Source: Adapted from National Institute for Health Research (2008).

The Royal College of Psychiatrists (2012) suggests that models of intensive community and crisis CAMHS share some common characteristics including:

- *Immediate response:* access a crisis response from a CAMHS professional within a few hours of initial request.
- *Out of hours cover*: able to respond within 24 hours 7 days a week, with cover provided by a professional who can undertake a mental health assessment at any hour.
- *Assertive engagement:* persistent approach with repeated attempts to make contact including immediate follow-up of young people who do not attend appointments.
- *Flexible approach*: safe meeting locations agreed with young person and or carer at a time that suits them.
- *Planned intensive intervention:* frequent clinical input including several contacts a week, and high staff to service user ratio until the need for intensive input is resolved.
- *Support the stepped care approach:* provide continuity of managed care to standard community, day or inpatient CAMHS care as required.
- *Collaborative relationships*: able to access other CAMHS professionals and agencies as required in order to meet the needs of the young person and their parents or carers.

Dialectical behaviour therapy

DBT was developed at the Behavioural Research and Therapy Clinics in the US by Linehan and colleagues (see Linehan 1993). Although developed as an outpatient treatment DBT can be used in both inpatient and forensic settings and probably deserves a chapter of its own. DBT has been adapted to use with young people, particularly those who repeatedly self-harm (Miller et al. 2007), and has been shown to be effective as an alternative to admission. It is increasingly being provided by specialist CAMHS across the UK.

DBT comprises a programme of individual and group therapy, social skills training and access to crisis management by telephone. Young people who are suicidal or self-harming often have multiple interpersonal problems and struggle to cope with strong emotions. Deciding where to start in making positive changes is often difficult for both the young person and their therapist. Like many other multi-modal treatment programmes DBT is highly structured. Treatment is organised in a four-stage hierarchy with targeted behaviours being addressed at one stage being brought under control before moving to the next stage (see Table 1.1).

DBT includes skills training at an individual and group level which comprises four modules. Whilst the mindfulness module is always completed first, subsequent modules on interpersonal effectiveness, emotional regulation and distress tolerance can be completed in any order (see Box 1.2).

Several RCTs have demonstrated that people who have used DBT have fewer suicidal ideas, are less likely to engage in para-suicidal behaviour and have fewer hospital admissions following self-harm (Koerner & Dimeff 2000; Dimeff et al. 2002; Katz et al. 2004). The National Institute for Clinical Excellence (NICE) guidelines on self-harm state that for people who self-harm and have a diagnosis of borderline personality disorder,

TABLE 1.1 DBT four-stage treatment hierarchy

Therapy stage	Focuses on
Pre-treatment	Assessment, commitment and orientation
1	Suicidal behaviours, therapy interfering behaviour, and behaviours that interfere with quality of life
2	Post-traumatic stress
3	Self esteem and individual treatment goals

BOX 1.2 DBT skills training group

Module 1	Mindfulness
Module 2	Interpersonal effectiveness
Module 3	Emotional regulation
Module 4	Distress tolerance

---

consideration should be given to the use of DBT (National Institute for Clinical Excellence 2004). DBT is also cited as an effective treatment in the NICE guidelines on the treatment and management of borderline personality disorder (National Collaborating Centre for Mental Health 2009).

What does the research tell us about effectiveness of hospital, intensive community and home-based services?

In contrast to research with adults, there is comparatively little research into alternatives to inpatient admission and home treatment for children and young people (Worrall-Davies & Kiernan, 2005). A review of the evidence undertaken by the National CAMHS support service on behalf of the Department of Health (Kurtz 2009) distilled a number of important findings in relation to Tier 4 CAMHS.

1 The effectiveness of interventions to meet what are typically complex, severe or persistent mental health problems in children and young people depends upon them being able to access the appropriate service, engaging with the therapeutic interventions that are on offer and staying with the treatment programme.

2 Interventions are likely to be more effective if they are provided early rather than late in a child's life course. This has implications for how we prioritise which services we offer and for whom they are provided. For example, some groups of children and young people are known to be at higher risk of mental health problems such as looked after children and young offenders.

3 Services are more effective if access to them is not dependent upon crisis situations but instead follow planned care pathways and a continuum of care for defined clinical needs.

4   Effectiveness depends on a full understanding of the needs of the child or young person. Before embarking on a programme of treatment or therapy a thorough assessment is required of what are invariably complex or entrenched needs. This process often takes time and cannot be addressed in a brief or superficial assessment.

5   In order to effectively address mental health problems and needs it is necessary to support the child or young person to tackle the problems that are causing most impairment or disability first. For example, young people need somewhere to live before you address their attachment problems. This has implications for how we prioritise treatment objectives and plan interventions.

6   Management of mental health problems is more effective if the child or young person's strengths and resilience are promoted. This again depends on knowing them well.

7   The delivery of effective interventions for children requiring hospital, intensive community and home-based services depends crucially on an appropriately trained, skilled and experienced workforce. Working with children and young people with complex psychosocial needs can be a challenging and emotionally draining process. It is therefore important that those providing care and treatment interventions have access to supervision and support from skilled practitioners.

8   It is important to measure outcomes across several domains. Improving functioning in one domain may have a positive effect in another. For example, treating a young person's attention deficit hyperactivity disorder (ADHD) may improve their educational attainment at school, or addressing a young person's depression may improve their social functioning. Measuring outcomes across domains also assists with multidisciplinary and multi-agency working, themselves crucial ingredients in work with young people who have complex psychosocial needs.

9   The difficulties young people are experiencing are often compounded by fragmented service provision. Single agency interventions are rarely effective, and can even be harmful as a range of needs may be neglected. There are only small numbers of jointly commissioned services for children and young people requiring intensive community services across the UK.

Similarly, in a review of the literature on intensive community and home-based programmes the Policy Research Bureau (2007) suggested that implementation is as important as programme content. Without good implementation and a focus on maintaining treatment fidelity, the Bureau claimed, the best planned interventions will fail. In their review of parenting interventions; home visiting programmes; multi systemic therapy; treatment foster care; and functional family therapy; the Policy Research Bureau point to a number of general principles that lead to effective implementation, and thus, effectiveness (see Box 1.3).

What does policy guidance say?

The NSF guidance on developing high quality multidisciplinary CAMHS teams summarises a number of good practice principles if services are to be effective (see Box 1.4).

More recently, government policy has suggested that the implementation of any evidence-based model requires careful design and strong project management and support,

---

BOX 1.3   Key features of effective programmes

All programmes should have a strong, coherent and clearly articulated evidence base.
All programmes should be delivered by professional, qualified and/or trained staff.
All programmes should have high treatment or model fidelity.
All programmes should be delivered in the young person's natural environment.
All programmes should be tailored to the needs of their core clientele.
All programmes should be multi-modal or multi-dimensional.
Partnership with families should be central to all programmes.
A tiered approach should be built into all programmes.
No intensive community or home-based programme is a quick fix.

Source: Policy Research Bureau (2007).

BOX 1.4   Key elements in a CAMHS service that works

- Strong inter-agency commitment over the medium to long-term, including a steering group or strategy group willing to tackle tricky issues, and a commitment to consulting with and acting on children's and families' views;
- Links with existing services within CAMHS, including the integration of the service within the CAMHS tiered framework and CAMHS development strategy;
- Links with other services and initiatives outside CAMHS e.g. education, the voluntary sector and area-based initiatives;
- An ability to attract new sources of funding;
- Retention of a stable, multidisciplinary staff group with opportunities for training and development;
- Positive commitment to continued evaluation and audit; and
- Balance between providing a direct service to users and influencing the broader network.

Source: Department of Health (2004).

---

especially in the early stages. The Department for Education guidance on delivering intensive interventions for looked after children and those on the edge of custody states that effective stakeholder engagement, both operationally and strategically, is a key to success (Department for Education 2011).

What do young people, parents and carers want?

The views of young people about hospital, intensive community and home-based services are discussed in detail later in this book. The Royal College of Psychiatrists (2012) have summarised views in relation to intensive crisis services in CAMHS and point out that young people and their carers want to:

- be reassured that help is available and immediately accessible, by the right professional at the right time;
- understand what is happening and receive information in a way that suits them;
- receive care in settings that are acceptable to the individual and their parent/carer;
- avoid admission if possible and receive intensive support in the community or at home;
- receive intensive support and continuity of care post-discharge from inpatient treatment to other services (facilitate stepped care).

There is also good evidence that the involvement of young people, parents and carers in care and treatment planning improves outcomes (Sourander et al. 1996; Grizenko 1997) and this is explored further in Chapter 10.

Summary

In the UK the 'tiered model' of service delivery remains the preferred framework to organise the commissioning, management and delivery of mental health services for children and young people with mental health problems and disorders. This is explored in some further detail in the next chapter.

Children and young people requiring hospital, intensive community or home-based services rarely respond to interventions that focus on them as individuals in isolation from the context in which they are living. The range of difficulties they are experiencing occur across multiple domains of functioning and require systemic and contextual understanding and multi-modal treatment strategies involving their family, school, social network and wider community. Not surprisingly, young people requiring hospital, intensive community or home-based services usually require multi-agency interventions. However, more research is needed to identify the component factors of intensive treatments which are effective and which distinguish one model or service from another.

A range of alternative services have been developed to manage some young people with complex mental health needs. These are in an outpatient, day care or other community setting. Such alternative services include assertive outreach, intensive community-based interventions, intensive treatment foster care, intensive outpatient or day services, and other specialist services. The Royal College of Psychiatrists (2006) suggests that intensive treatment can be developed as the result of collaboration between specialist CAMHS and social services or education or all three of these, through joint work between Tier 3 and Tier 4 CAMHS or collaboration between specialist CAMHS and paediatrics or CAMHS and adult mental health. However, this range of hospital, intensive community and home-based services that national policy recommends and research has shown to be effective have, on the whole, not been developed in all parts of the UK. Some are described in the chapters in this book.

The NSF sets the expectation that there is an evidence-based approach to practice which presents a particular challenge to professionals working in CAMHS. Although there is an increasing volume of robust research on the effectiveness of mental health interventions with children and young people, there are a number of limitations to the current research base for CAMHS in the UK. Children and young people rarely present with single disorders but rather with a range of difficulties. A large proportion of the available evidence does not reflect the complexity and comorbidity that is often part of day to day clinical practice. Consequently, the interventions we are using in hospital, intensive community and home-based services have often not been tested in research.

This, however, does not necessarily mean that the interventions we are using are ineffective. Rather, it may indicate that more research is needed to determine its effectiveness or otherwise. The small evidence base focused on hospital, intensive community and home-based interventions tells us that fidelity to model is important. Manualised and multi-modal treatment strategies are evidence based and it is vital that we preserve these models over time to evaluate longer-term outcomes.

It is important for the work of hospital, intensive community and home-based services to be properly monitored and evaluated and the information used to enhance clinical work, to further service development and to inform users and other stakeholders. It is clear that we need more research about which service models work for children and young people with severe, complex or persistent mental disorders who have not responded to intervention at Tier 3 CAMHS level. This requires collaboration between multi-agency commissioners, service providers and researchers. This partnership is essential to supply the evidence on which future clinical and commissioning decisions can be made and services can be provided.

References

Burns BJ, Costello EJ, Angold A, Tweed D, et al. (1995). Children's mental health service use across service sectors. *Health Affairs* 14,147–60.

Byford S, Barrett B, Roberts C, Clark A, Edwards V, Harrington R, Smethurst N, Gowers S. (2007). Economic evaluation of a randomised controlled treatment trial for adolescent anorexia nervosa. *British Journal of Psychiatry* 191,436–40.

Department for Children, Schools and Families. (2008). *Children and Young People in Mind: the final report of the National CAMHS Review*. London: HMSO.

Department for Education. (2011). *Prospectus: delivering intensive interventions for looked after children and those on the edge of custody and their families*. London: HMSO.

Department of Health. (2012). *Clinical Advisory Group for Prescribed Services: final recommendations*. London: HMSO.

Department of Health. (2004). *National Service Framework for Children, Young People and Maternity Services*. London: HMSO.

Dimeff L, Koerner K, Linehan M. (2002). Summary of research on dialectical behaviour therapy. *Clinical Psychology, Science and Practice* 7, 104–112.

Evans M, Boothroyd R, Armstrong M, Greenbaum P, Brown E, Kuppinger A. (2003). An experimental study of the effectiveness of intensive in-home crisis services for children and their families: program outcomes. *Journal of Emotional and Behavioral Disorders* 11(2), 92–121.

Gowers SG, Clark A, Roberts A, Griffiths A, Edwards V, Bryan C, Smethurst N, Byford S, Barrett B. (2007). Clinical effectiveness of treatments for anorexia nervosa in adolescents: randomised controlled trial. *British Journal of Psychiatry*. 191, 427–435.

Green J, Worrall-Davies A. (2008). Provision of intensive treatment: in-patient units, day units and intensive outreach. In: Rutter M, Bishop D, Pine D, Scott S, Stevenson J, Taylor E, Thapar A (Eds). *Child and Adolescent Psychiatry*, 5th edition. Blackwell Publishing.

Grizenko N. (1997) Outcome of a multi-modal day treatment for children with severe behaviour problems: a five-year follow-up. *Journal of the American Academy of Child and Adolescent Psychiatry* 36, 989–997.

Grizenko N, Papineau D, Sayegh L. (1993a). A comparison of day treatment and outpatient treatment for children with disruptive behavior problems. *Canadian Journal of Psychiatry* 38, 432–435.

Grizenko N, Papineau D, Sayegh L. (1993b). Effectiveness of a multimodal day treatment program for children with disruptive behavior problems. *Journal of American Academy of Child and Adolescent Psychiatry* 32, 127–134.

Hearnshaw H. (2004). Comparison of requirements of research ethics committees in 11 European countries for a non invasive interventional study, *British Medical Journal* 328, 140–141.

Henggeler SW, Rowland MD, Randall J, Ward DM, Pickrel SG, Cunningham PB, Miller S, Edwards J, Zealberg JJ, Hand LE, Santos AB. (1999). Home-based multisystemic therapy as an alternative to the hospitalisation of youths in psychiatric crisis: clinical outcomes. *Journal of American Academy of Child and Adolescent Psychiatry*, 38(11), 1331–1339.

House of Commons. (2001). *The Report of the Royal Liverpool Children's Inquiry.* London: HMSO.

Katz L, Cox B, Gunasekara S, Miller A. (2004). Feasibility of dialectical behaviour therapy for suicidal adolescent patients. *Journal of the American Academy of Child and Adolescent Psychiatry* 43(3), 276–282.

Koerner K, Dimeff L. (2000). Further data on dialectical behaviour therapy. *Clinical Psychology Science and Practice* 7, 104–112.

Kurtz, Z (2007). *Regional Review of Tier 4 Child and Adolescent Mental Health Services.* London: Department of Health.

Kurtz, Z. (2009). *The Evidence Base to Guide Development of Tier 4 CAMHS.* London: HMSO.

Lamb C. (2009). Alternatives to admission for children and adolescents: providing intensive mental healthcare services at home and in communities: what works? *Current Opinion in Psychiatry* 22(4), 345–350.

Linehan, M. (1993). *Skills Training Manual for Treating Borderline Personality Disorder.* New York: Guilford.

Littell JH, Popa M, Forsythe B. (2005). Multisystemic Therapy for social, emotional, and behavioral problems in youth aged 10-17. *Cochrane Database of Systematic Reviews* Issue 4. Art. No.: CD004797. DOI: 10.1002/14651858.

McDougall, T. (2006). *Child and Adolescent Mental Health Nursing.* London: Blackwell.

McDougall T, Worrall-Davies A, Hewson L, Richardson G, Cotgrove A. (2008). Tier 4 Child and Adolescent Mental Health Services: inpatient care, day services and alternatives: an overview of Tier 4 CAMHS provision in the UK. *Child and Adolescent Mental Health*, 13(4), 173–180.

Mattejat F, Hirt BR, Wilkem J, Schmidt MH, Remeschmidt H. (2001) Efficacy of inpatient and home treatment in psychiatrically disturbed children and adolescents: follow up assessment of the results of a controlled treatment study. *European Journal of Child and Adolescent Psychiatry* 10(1), 171–179.

Meenaghan A, O'Herlih, A, Durand M, Farr H, Tulloch S, Lelliott P. (2007). A 55kg paper mountain: the impact of new research governance and ethics processes on mental health services research in England. *Journal of Mental Health* 16(1), 149–155.

Miller A, Rathus J, Linehan M. (2007). *Dialectical Behavior Therapy with Suicidal Adolescents.* New York: Guilford Press.

National Collaborating Centre for Mental Health. (2009). *Borderline Personality Disorder: treatment and management.* National Clinical Guideline Number 78. London: NICE.

National Institute for Clinical Excellence. (2004). *The Short Term Physical and Psychological Management and Secondary Prevention of Self Harm in Primary and Secondary Care.* National Clinical Practice Guideline Number 16. London: NICE.

National Institute for Health Research. (2009). *Research Summary: alternatives to inpatient care for children and adolescents with complex mental health needs.* London: NIHR.

NHS Health Advisory Service. (1995). *Together we Stand: the commissioning, role and management of child and adolescent mental health services*. London: HMSO.

Pecora P, Fraser M, Bennett R, Haapala D. (1991). Placement rates of children and families served by intensive family preservation services program. In: Fraser M, Pecora P, Haapala D. (Eds). *Families in Crisis*. New York: Aldine.

Policy Research Bureau. (2007). *Interventions for Children at Risk of Developing Antisocial Personality Disorder: report to the Department of Health and Prime Minister's Strategy Unit*. London: Policy Research Bureau.

Rowland M, Halliday-Boykins C, Henggeler S, Cunningham P, Lee T, Krusei M, Shapiro S. (2005). A randomised trial of multi systemic therapy with Hawaii's Felix class youth. *Journal of Emotional and Behavioral Disorders* 13(1), 13–23.

Royal College of Psychiatrists. (2006). *Building and Sustaining Specialist Child and Adolescent Mental Health Services*. London: RCP.

Royal College of Psychiatrists. (2012).*Quality Network for Community CAMHS*. London: CCQI.

Schmidt M, Lay B, Gopel C, Naab S, Blanz B. (2006). Home treatment for children and adolescents with psychiatric disorders. *European Child & Adolescent Psychiatry* 15, 265–276.

Schwartz I, Wernert T. (1993). Reducing psychiatric hospitalisation for children and adolescent in Toledo, Ohio: community alternatives. *International Journal of Family Care* 5(2), 71–78.

Shetty P. (2007). Mental health services for children patchy in the UK. *The Lancet* 370(9582), 123–124.

Sourander A, Turunen MM. (1999). Psychiatric hospital care among children and adolescents in Finland: a nationwide register study. *Social Psychiatry and Psychiatric Epidemiology* 34, 105–110.

Sourander A, Helenius H, Leijala H, Heikkilae T, Bergroth L, Piha J. (1996). Predictors of outcome of short-term child psychiatric inpatient treatment. *European Journal of Child and Adolescent Psychiatry* 5, 75–82.

Thomsen PH. (1996). A 22- to 25-year follow-up study of former child psychiatric patients: a register-based investigation of the course of psychiatric disorder and mortality in 546 Danish child psychiatric patients. *Acta Psychiatrica Scandinavica* 94, 397–403.

Wilmshurst L. (2002). Treatment programs for youth with emotional and behavioural disorders: an outcome study of two alternative approaches. *Mental Health Services Research* 4(2): 85–96.

Winsberg B, Bialer I, Kupietz S, Botti E, Balka E. (1980). Home vs hospital care of children with behaviour disorders. *Archives of General Psychiatry* 37, 413–418.

Woolston, J. (1998). Intensive, integrated, in-home psychiatric services: the catalyst to enhancing out-patient intervention. *Child and Adolescent Psychiatric Clinics of North America*, 7(3), 615–633.

Worrall-Davies A, Kiernan K. (2005). *Using a Virtual Team: an evaluation of the Bradford CAMHS intensive home treatment approach*. Leeds: Bradford Children and Young People's Partnership. University of Leeds.

York A. Lamb C. (2005). *Building and Sustaining Specialist CAMHS: workforce, capacity and functions of Tiers 2, 3, and 4 Specialist Child and Adolescent Mental Health Services across England, Ireland, Northern Ireland, Scotland and Wales*. London: Royal College of Psychiatrists.

2

REFERRAL PATHWAYS INTO HOSPITAL, INTENSIVE COMMUNITY AND HOME-BASED SERVICES

Tim McDougall and Andy Cotgrove

Key points

- When describing the range of hospital, intensive community and home-based services that are required it is helpful to separate the core functions of managing high risk and providing intensive interventions that cannot be provided cost-effectively or with sufficient expertise in local teams. Consideration should also be given to the services that agencies provide so that young people do not enter the wrong pathway or end up in the wrong service.
- Factors leading to referral to Tier 4 CAMHS are not only the severity and complexity of the child or young person's mental disorder, but also lack of treatment response, unusual clinical features, breakdown in therapeutic relationships, unavailability of local treatment options, increased vulnerability due to personal circumstances and patient choice.
- The only criteria for unplanned admission should be those young people presenting with high risk due to mental health difficulties who cannot be managed safely in the community. There are no other indications for an unplanned admission.
- The process of planning discharge should occur even before a child or young person is admitted to hospital or accepted by intensive community services. Good discharge planning by the Tier 4 team will involve the establishment of regular communication with referrers, clarification of their ongoing involvement and exploration of the possibility of joint interventions whilst the child or young person is receiving Tier services.
- In order to facilitate clear pathways of care some organisations have developed transition support and outreach teams to strengthen links between Tier 3 and 4 services and facilitate the process of admission and discharge from hospital. Outreach and transition support services have been successful in reducing length of stay and preventing readmission to hospital. However, their clinical and cost-effectiveness need closer examination.

Introduction

When thinking about what services and pathways are needed in Tier 4 CAMHS, a good starting principle is that 'form' should follow 'function'. The core function of Tier 4 CAMHS is arguably to manage and treat young people who:

1   present with high-risk behaviours associated with mental disorders, and/or;
2   need high intensity interventions that cannot be provided cost-effectively or with sufficient expertise in local teams such as Tier 3 CAMHS.

The form with which this function can be delivered is various. Historically Tier 4 services have been based on inpatient beds, but increasingly it is recognised that the functions of Tier 4 can be achieved by providing a range of hospital, intensive community and home-based services. In this chapter an outline is given of how young people may reach Tier 4 services, and what options are available to meet their needs within the available resources. Details about some of the component parts of Tier 4 services are discussed further throughout the book.

Who gets referred to hospital, intensive community and home-based services?

There has only been very limited research on why children and young people are referred to hospital, intensive community and home-based services, the reasons they are accepted or admitted, the treatments they receive and their pathways following discharge. With the exception of a small number of multi-site studies (Wrate et al. 1994; O'Herlihy et al. 2007) reports are clinical descriptions and reflect the experience of single service providers.

Factors leading to referral to Tier 4 CAMHS are not only the severity and complexity of the child or young person's mental disorder, but also lack of treatment response, unusual clinical features, breakdown in therapeutic relationships, unavailability of local treatment options, increased vulnerability due to personal circumstances and patient choice (Department of Health 2012). Inequity in provision, service and organisational factors are also likely to influence referral and admission decisions. This has been shown to be true in the US where admission thresholds differ according to the level of resources available (Bickman et al. 1996).

Indeed, this has been found to be true in the UK where an unpublished study of referrals to an inpatient adolescent service quadrupled when the option of emergency access for referrers became available (McDougall 2012). In her review of Tier 4 services in England, Kurtz (2007) stresses that the type of intervention and care that needs to be carried out within a psychiatric inpatient setting requires clearer definition. She suggests that patterns of admission are strongly influenced by what is available in day patient, outpatient, outreach and community-based services; pointing out that the existence of these kinds of services is patchy, both geographically and in terms of the expertise and facilities they provide. The Royal College of Psychiatrists (2006) go as far as to suggest that the capacity and capability of Tier 3 largely defines what Tier 4 is.

A common set of indicators for hospital admission has not been agreed among researchers and clinicians, but for the minority that do need admission, there are a number of common denominators. According to the Royal College of Psychiatrists (2008) these include:

- a degree of risk to self or others that cannot safely be managed in the community;
- intransigent family difficulties making home or community treatment difficult;
- the need for 24-hour supervision and nursing care.

Some clinicians place greater emphasis on the use of hospital admission to clarify diagnosis in a 'controlled environment' (Wrate et al. 1994; Green 2002) but there is some disagreement on this point.

One obvious solution to clarify referral pathways is to define clear service boundaries. However, this is not without problems. Kurtz (2007) suggests that it should not be seen as desirable to draw exact boundaries between Tier 3 and Tier 4 but to define the elements of these specialist services that should be available, with the skills and resources attached, and how they should integrate with each other to meet the continuum of young people's needs.

Most referrals to most Tier 4 services are made by professionals in Tier 3 CAMHS. A guiding principle for referral to Tier 4 should be that the young person's needs cannot be managed safely or effectively within a lower tiered service. This is because only those young people with the greatest needs should be referred to the most intensive level of service provision. There are a range of complex factors that affect the composition and resources of Tier 3 CAMHS and referrals to Tier 4 services are often determined by what can be managed by the community team (Department of Health 2009).

Young people with mental health needs may come to the attention of services in a variety of ways, and not necessarily in the way that best addresses their needs. For example, a young person suffering from abuse or neglect may present to social care because they have run away from home; to mental health services because they are self-harming; or to the police because they have acted antisocially or broken the law. With a lack of integration between these services the young person may enter a system that only addresses the problem they present with and does not get their underlying or holistic needs met in the most appropriate way.

Shepherd (2006) illustrates this concern from the perspective of education. Whilst young people with a statement of special educational needs (SEN) might be placed in a residential special school to meet their educational needs, their health, social care needs and possibly safeguarding issues may have been overlooked. Despite regulations that are designed to ensure notification to other agencies, Shepherd points out that young people are often placed without the receiving authority being aware of the young person's needs. This potential for fragmentation of care applies across all services and in all agencies. However, with appropriate assessment, and good multi-agency working this fragmentation in care can be overcome.

What are the pathways to Tier 4 services?

The concept of 'pathways to care' offers a way of exploring the use of health resources (O'Herlihy et al. 2007). So what do the right pathways look like and which services are needed? The Royal College of Psychiatrists (2006) suggests that Tier 4 services are an integral part of overall CAMHS delivery and depend on good relationships with successful community and multi-agency services. They propose that a close working relationship between Tier 3 and Tier 4 CAMHS is fundamental to the delivery of an effective comprehensive CAMHS service. CAMHS cannot be considered safe or comprehensive if it does not have access to specialist adolescent inpatient facilities offering the option of emergency admissions for children and young people with severe mental illness and associated risks. This interdependency between community and inpatient services is discussed further in the next chapter and the referral pathways into a range of intensive community and home-based services are discussed throughout this book.

Gaps in pathways and access

On the basis that the form of these services should follow the function, the model of care for Tier 4 should include crisis assessment and management services, planned intensive home treatment services, and hospital beds for those that require them. Each of these elements are of too 'low volume' to justify local commissioning but can provide alternatives to admission for many children and young people. When there are gaps in multi-agency service provision, it can result in young people being 'stuck' at the wrong level on a pathway or on the wrong pathway altogether.

Street (2000) highlights a number of gaps in access to Tier 4 CAMHS including long-erm therapeutic provision and post-discharge support services which lead to an over-dependence on inpatient CAMHS and increased numbers of emergency referrals. Intensive community services such as treatment foster care and multisystemic therapy are not available in all areas of the UK, and where gaps in access exist, young people with complex psychosocial needs may receive the wrong service or face a long wait for the right service.

If the commissioners of Tier 4 only provide beds this is all that young people with high levels of need will get. A bed-based model of care will also inevitably result in more admissions than are necessary. For example, a review of Tier 4 CAMHS commissioning in London in 2008 found serious gaps in provision with a high reliance on 'spot purchasing' from the independent sector. Additionally, the review found a lack of strategic planning and a lack of basic information about care patterns, cost of provision and monitoring (Banton 2008). This finding was supported by the CAMHS Inpatient Referral Study (CIRS) which found that the great majority of young people who are denied admission to an NHS unit and are then referred on, are subsequently admitted to an independent sector unit (O'Herlihy et al. 2007).

Admission or acceptance into hospital, intensive community or home-based services

Guidance on inpatient CAMHS points out that admission must operate within a pathway of care, involving the local community teams. This is essential to avoid a protracted length of stay or care episode; the development of dependency on inpatient treatment; and loss of contact by the young person with their family and community (Department of Health 2009). These principles apply equally to intensive community and home-based services. Corbett and Evans (2002) suggest that effective use of specialist Tier 4 provision is dependent on the development of care pathways, led by local CAMHS teams. These need to be designed to ensure timely referral to Tier 4, with local involvement in the process of admission and in care planning during admission to facilitate transition back into the community with support from local services.

According to Maskey (1998), referrals for inpatient treatment fall into three categories. First are 'enquiries', where the referrer is uncertain about the need for inpatient treatment or if the unit would be able to meet the young person's needs. Second are actual 'referrals', where the referrer is confident about the need for admission and anticipates that the unit will be able to meet the young person's needs. Third are 'emergencies' where the referral is made in crisis.

All three types of referrals require an assessment before decisions about admission or acceptance into service are made. This is because Tier 4 services are intensive and intrusive, particularly inpatient admission. We must be fairly confident that it will not make things worse rather than better for young people. It is therefore important for both referrers and assessors to carefully consider the relative costs as well as benefits of a Tier 4 intervention. Lincoln and McGorry (1995) emphasise the need to examine care pathways beyond the 'gateway'. They suggest employing a model that can consider the impact on the lives of those affected and how their future care paths are shaped.

The numbers of children and young people with complex, severe or persistent mental disorders and an associated level of risk which cannot be managed safely at Tier 3 should be few rather than many. Therefore, a comprehensive and well functioning Tier 3 team will keep referrals to Tier 4 to a minimum. At some point, however, the complexity, severity or risk of an individual young person will necessitate a referral to Tier 4, whether this is an intensive community, home-based or inpatient service.

The 'low volume' nature of hospital, intensive community and home-based services means that it is inefficient for them to be developed in Tier 3 or across single local authority footprints. Hence Tier 4 services are commissioned and provided across a larger footprint so they can develop expertise in providing more intensive services for a larger number of young people. This is also why proposals to develop so-called 'Tier 3½', 'Tier 3 plus' or 'enhanced Tier 3' services have been unhelpful and have arguably contributed to an historic neglect of Tier 4 commissioning.

Planned referrals

To avoid inappropriate or unnecessary Tier 4 interventions it is usually preferable for Tier 4 clinicians to be involved in a joint assessment prior to admission. The only criteria for unplanned admission should be those young people presenting with high risk due to mental health difficulties who cannot be managed safely in the community. There are no other indications for an unplanned admission. Avoiding unnecessary admissions allows for a more thorough, planned assessment of a young persons needs. For many young people, once their crisis has subsided, their needs may be met by services outside Tier 4 CAMHS, and often within Tier 3. However, for those who have complex difficulties requiring a specialist or intensity of intervention not available elsewhere, treatment within Tier 4 is indicated. These needs may be met by a planned admission, but alternatives to this can also be considered that would not be available in a Tier 3 service. The ways in which clinicians can plan admissions collaboratively with young people and parents is discussed in the next chapter.

Unplanned referrals

When making a referral for Tier 4 services it is important that there is clarity about what is required. Often, young people are referred because it is clear that they are in a high state of distress and they need to be kept safe. It is often unclear immediately what needs to change to alter this position and how Tier 4 services can help enable that change.

Inappropriate unplanned admissions should be avoided for several reasons. First, there is evidence that services to support young people are more effective if access to them is not dependent upon crisis situations (Massie et al. 2008). Second, outcomes are better when admissions have clear objectives. And third, admissions can be harmful, for example by removing the young person from their family, friends, school and other social support; or by reinforcing and escalating unhelpful coping strategies such as self-harm (Dalton et al. 1989; Green & Jones 1998; Jaffa & Stott 1999; Bobier & Warwick 2004). In addition, hospital admissions are costly and not necessarily the best use of the scarce resources in Tier 4 services.

In highlighting the unintended consequences of an inpatient admission, Green and Jones (1998) warn of the loss of local professional involvement where local agencies may take admission as a cue to withdraw completely from involvement in a child or young person's care. Commenting on the reasons for hospital admission, the Scottish Executive (2005) points out that a young people's psychiatric inpatient unit cannot replace good quality social work services or fill the gap in local child and adolescent mental health services.

Emergency referrals

The Royal College of Psychiatrists (2006) suggests that there are three main types of problems that young people experience which often present as emergencies:

1   Where there is an identified serious mental health problem, for example, psychosis, depression, serious risk of self-harm and, rarely, very serious eating disorder. For the latter, the risk may be due to physical deterioration and require medical admission.
2   Young people presenting to a general hospital ward via accident and emergency department following an episode of self-harm. The treatment needs are less clear in this group and in most cases admission to a paediatric ward followed by assessment and follow up by Tier 2 or 3 CAMHS is appropriate.
3   Children and adolescents with conduct disorders, out of control and challenging behaviour, where there is often inter-agency confusion and disagreement about what is needed to help.

The ideal pathway for a young person in crisis presenting with high-risk behaviour requires:

1   CAMHS clinicians available 24 hours a day with relevant experience to assess which young people require immediate admissions;

2   access to age appropriate beds 24 hours a day;
3   access to non-bed-based alternatives in the community to manage high levels of risk
     as an alternative to admission.

Where one or more of these three core components are not available the potential for inappropriate hospital admission is increased.

Admission avoidance services

There is some learning for CAMHS from the experience of adult services. As well as beds, adult mental health services have crisis resolution and home treatment teams (Department of Health, 1999). These are designed to assess people in crisis and determine the most appropriate intervention. This may include admission or intensive home treatment. Implementing this model over the last 10 years has resulted in substantial reductions in the need for admissions, improved patient experience and freed up resources for community services. Although crises are rarer in young people, the same principles apply, and crisis resolution and home treatment services for young people would help to avoid inappropriate and potentially harmful admissions.

The Royal College of Psychiatrists (2012) has suggested that non-bed-based CAMHS crisis and intensive service models have developed in response to:

• an ideological move away from residential psychiatric care, and a need to offer alternative options of intensive care;
• recognition of the chronicity and long-term mental health pathways followed by some young people with severe, persistent and complex needs;
• a need to provide options of care more acceptable to young people, encompassing their family and wider community.

Duffy & Skeldon (2012) report that a CAMHS intensive treatment service, with close links to an adolescent inpatient unit, can provide a balanced care approach where young people with severe mental health difficulties can be treated in the community, where possible, without compromising patient safety and quality of care. Similarly, Darwish and colleagues (2006) describe a community intensive therapy team (CITT) which has been operating since 1998. It was developed to cater for the needs of young people with complex difficulties comparable with young people who might be referred for admission to an inpatient unit. These include those with eating disorders, psychosis, affective disorders, adjustment disorders and repetitive self-harm. Since its inception, the CITT has been able to manage all the complex referrals made to it from the generic Tier 2 and 3 CAMHS teams with minimal recourse to inpatient beds.

Discharge

The process of planning discharge should occur even before a young person is admitted to hospital or accepted by an intensive community team. Good discharge planning by the

Tier 4 service will involve the establishment of regular communication with referrers, clarification of their ongoing involvement and exploration of the possibility of joint interventions whilst the child or young person is in hospital or community treatment.

As a prelude to discharge from inpatient care a 'stepped care' model may facilitate safe and timely discharge whereby more nights are spent at home or in day services. By offering inpatient, day patient or outpatient programmes more flexibly, children and young people can be offered a staged discharge (Department of Health 2009). This flexible arrangement allows the child or young person to return to hospital if they deteriorate, and when it may be necessary to work more intensively. It promotes a collaborative approach with young people and their families and enables the multidisciplinary and multi-agency team to tailor treatment packages for each individual.

Recognising that children and young people move in and out of need and are not simply on a trajectory, the National Advisory Council recommended that 'step down' services to support managed moves from specialist provision to less intensive services should be available for children and young people (Department for Children, Schools and Families 2008). In order to facilitate clear pathways of care some organisations have developed transition support and outreach teams to strengthen links between Tier 3 and 4 services and facilitate the process of admission, discharge and young people transitioning to adult or community services. For example, the Chester Assessment and Outreach Team (AOT) is a small nurse-led service that fulfils three functions:

1   gate-keeps admission to Tier 4 beds;
2   provides outreach to facilitate timely discharge;
3   prevents admission by working with young people intensively in the community.

Another service is the CAMHS Outreach and Therapies Service (CO&TS) in Leeds. This is an intensive community service working with families with specific needs which cannot be fully met in Tier 3. CO&TS aims to prevent admission to, and enable early discharge from, the local inpatient service by providing intensive community support. However, where clinically indicated, outreach and therapeutic input is provided by the inpatient team.

The outcomes of outreach and other admission avoidance services have not been widely reported and systematic research is required to determine their cost and clinical effectiveness.

Young people with complex psychosocial needs

One group of young people who are at particular risk of entering services arbitrarily is those with complex psychosocial needs. Whilst the needs of young people in this group are not homogeneous, a number of common factors commonly unite them. They often have backgrounds characterised by high levels of psychosocial adversity and may have suffered from substantial trauma, abuse and loss. Due to poor family functioning and breakdown, young people with complex psychosocial needs may have experienced numerous and disrupted care placements. This group with complex psychosocial needs includes young people:

- with poor attachments and complex needs, whose severe and persistent behaviour problems are out of control in mainstream or intensive children's services;
- who engage in serious self-harm and who are not motivated to stop self-harming;
- whose oppositional, aggressive or violent behaviour places other people at risk.

Despite their heterogeneity, young people with complex psychosocial needs have a number of common characteristics that cluster them together for the purposes of commissioning and providing services. At any one time, research suggests that there are two or three young people per local authority who are the most challenging to look after and the most difficult to place in services (Clark et al. 2005). Their needs are 'high cost–low volume' and often require bespoke multi-modal care and treatment strategies. These are to provide physical and psychological containment, individual and family interventions and social skills building. Interventions include those targeted towards:

- poor family functioning and breakdown;
- risk to self through self-harm or high-risk behaviour;
- risk from others arising from vulnerability to abuse and exploitation;
- risk to others through violence;
- interrupting pathways to offending;
- emerging borderline and antisocial personality disorder;
- drug and alcohol interventions;
- psychosexual education.

Perhaps not surprisingly, young people with complex psychosocial needs are at heightened risk of poor transitions as their needs span more than one agency and numerous services. Whether a young person is placed in a social care or health setting will make a difference to long-term outcomes. However, routes in and out of community and residential care in social care and health establishments are somewhat arbitrary. Some young people who require inpatient or residential care and treatment remain in the community whereas others who require community interventions are admitted or accommodated inappropriately. Others may spiral through the care system and may be placed in independent sector intensive residential services or secure accommodation. Some may reach intensive community or home-based services appropriately, whereas others are admitted to hospital inappropriately. A proportion enters the youth justice system when their aggressive, antisocial or offending behaviour involves them breaking the law. The multi-agency costs of supporting young people with complex psychosocial needs is highly variable, often with no discernible relationship between care pathways, problems and needs, placement specification and outcomes for the young people concerned.

Future pathways

Pathways to care are becoming more sophisticated. For example, as part of the recognition, detection, risk profiling and referral of children and young people with depression (NCCMH 2005) the National Institute for Health and Care Excellence has developed a clinical pathway. This includes referral to Tier 4 CAMHS if the child or young person with depression has one or more of the following features:

- high recurrent risks of acts of self-harm or suicide;
- significant ongoing neglect (such as poor personal hygiene or significant reduction in eating that could be harmful to physical health);
- requirement for intensity of assessment/treatment and/or level of supervision that is not available in Tier 2 or 3.

As other NICE guidelines are developed that address mental health disorders affecting children and young people it is likely that they will also include clinical pathways. In turn, these may influence which children and young people get referred to Tier 4 services and at what stage. Combined, these pathways may contribute to better strategic planning and delivery of intensive community, home-based and hospital-based services.

Summary

The development of coherent referral pathways for young people requiring hospital, intensive community and home-based services is the responsibility of commissioners and local strategic partnerships of providers. Ensuring young people follow the right pathways of course depends on a range of services being available to meet the young person's needs across several domains.

The appropriate role and the effectiveness of Tier 4 services depend crucially upon integrated working with local Tier 3 CAMHS. To ensure young people are helped at the right level and at the right time it is essential that the key agencies in health, social care, education and youth justice all work together to help ensure a young person with multiple and complex needs receives the most appropriate interventions.

References

Banton, R. (2008). *London Child and Adolescent Mental Health Service Tier 4 Inpatient Commissioning Review*. London: NHS London Specialised Commissioning Group.

Bickman, L., Foster, E.M. & Lambert, E.W. (1996). Who gets hospitalized in a continuum of care? *Journal of the American Academy of Child and Adolescent Psychiatry*, 35(1), 74–80.

Bobier, C. & Warwick, M. (2004). Factors associated with readmission to adolescent psychiatric care. *Australian and New Zealand Journal of Psychiatry*, 39, 600–606.

Clark, A., O'Malley, A. & Woodham, A. (2005). Children with complex mental health problems: needs, costs and predictors over 1 year. *Child and Adolescent Mental Health*, 10(4), 170–178.

Corbett, K. & Evans, M. (2002) *Improving Child and Adolescent Mental Health Services in the West Midlands. Tier 4 CAMHS, A Strategy for Consultation. West Midlands.* Birmingham: National Institute of Mental Health for England.

Dalton, R., Muller, B. & Forman, M. (1989). The psychiatric hospitalization of children: an overview. *Child Psychiatry and Human Development*, 19(4), 231–244.

Darwish, A., Salmon, G., Ahuja, A. & Steed, L. (2006). The community intensive therapy team: development and philosophy of a new service. *Clinical Child Psychology and Psychiatry*, 11(4), 591–605.

Department for Children, Schools and Families. (2008). *Children and Young People in Mind: the final report of the National CAMHS Review*. London: HMSO.

Department of Health. (2012). *Clinical Advisory Group for Prescribed Services: final recommendations*. London: HMSO.

Department of Health. (2009). *Working within Child and Adolescent Inpatient Services: a practitioners handbook by Angela Sergeant*. London: HMSO.

Department of Health. (1999). *National Service Framework for Mental Heath*. London: HMSO.

Duffy, F. & Skeldon, J. (2012). A CAMHS intensive treatment service: clinical outcomes in the first year. *Clinical Child Psychology and Psychiatry*, doi: 10.1177/1359104512468287.

Green, J. (2002). Provision of intensive treatment: Inpatient units, day units and intensive outreach. In: Rutter, M. & Taylor, E. (Eds). *Child and Adolescent Psychiatry*. London: Blackwell Publishing, 1038–1050.

Green, J. & Jones, D. (1998). Unwanted effects of inpatient treatment: anticipation, prevention and repair. In: Green, J. & Jacobs, B. (Eds). *Inpatient Psychiatry: modern practice, research and the future*. London: Routledge.

Jaffa, T. & Stott, C. (1999). Do inpatients on adolescent units recover? A study of outcome and acceptability of treatment. *European Child and Adolescent Psychiatry*, 8, 292–300.

Kurtz, Z. (2007). *Regional Reviews of Tier 4 Child and Adolescent Mental Health Services*. London: HMSO.

Lincoln, C. & McGorry, P. (1995). Who cares? Pathways to psychiatric care for young people experiencing a first episode of psychosis. *Psychiatric Services*, 46(11), 1166–1171.

Maskey, S. (1998). The process of admission. In: Green, J. & Jacobs, B. (Eds). *Inpatient Psychiatry: modern practice, research and the future*. London: Routledge.

Massie, L. (2008). Right time, right place: Learning from the Children's national Service Framework development initiatives for psychological wellbeing and mental health, 2005-2007 http://www.chimat.org.uk/resource/item.aspx?RID=85818.

McDougall, T. (2012). *First 100 Referrals to an Inpatient Adolescent Unit: the role of the assessment and outreach team*. Unpublished paper. Cheshire and Wirral Foundation NHS Trust.

National Collaborating Centre for Mental Health (2005) *Depression in Children and Young People: identification and management in primary, community and secondary care*. National Clinical Practice Guideline Number 28. London. NICE.

O'Herlihy, A., Lelliott, P., Cotgrove, A., Andiappan, M. & Farr, H. (2007). *The Care Paths of Young People Referred But Not Admitted to Inpatient Child and Adolescent Mental Health Services*. London: Department of Health.

Royal College of Psychiatrists. (2006). *Building and Sustaining Specialist Child and Adolescent Mental Health Services*. Council Report 137. London: RCP.

Royal College of Psychiatrists. (2008). *The Costs, Outcomes and Satisfaction for Inpatient Child and Adolescent Psychiatric Services (COSI-CAPS) Study*. London: RCP.

Royal College of Psychiatrists. (2012). *Quality Network for Community CAMHS*. London: CCQI.

Scottish Executive. (2005). *Child Health Support Group: Inpatient Working Group Psychiatric Inpatient Services for Children and Young People in Scotland: a way forward*. http://www.scotland.gov.uk/Publications/2005/01/20523/49969

Shepherd, J. (2006). Commissioning for complex needs across agencies. In: Tier 4 CAMHS: *Improving, Expanding and Reforming: report of a conference by the National CAMHS Support Service and the Department of Health*. London: HMSO.

Street, C. (2000). *Whose crisis? Meeting the needs of children and young people with serious mental health problems*. London: Young Minds.

Wrate, R., Rothery, D., McCabe, R., Aspin, J. & Bryce, G. (1994). A prospective multi centre study of admissions to adolescent psychiatry inpatient units. *Journal of Adolescence*, 17, 221–237.

3

INPATIENT SERVICES

Andy Cotgrove

Key points

- Inpatient services should be provided as one part of a CAMHS pathway alongside other non-bed-based Tier 4 services.
- Criteria should be established for inpatient admission based on risk and complexity.
- Outcomes will be improved if clear aims are agreed with the young person and their families or carers prior to admission.
- Admission carries risks as well as potential benefits which need to be considered when agreeing with a referrer whether or not to admit a young person.
- Inpatient units should provide a range of individual, group and family interventions and have expertise in prescribing medications.
- The future is likely to see an increase in services designed to prevent avoidable admissions, intensive community-based alternatives to admission and a continuation of the current trend to separate acute inpatient beds from planned treatment beds. These areas should be seen as commissioning priorities within Tier 4 CAMHS.

Introduction

This chapter focuses on the role of inpatient units within the range of specialist child and adolescent mental health services (CAMHS). Historically, inpatient units were the main way of delivering services to young people with complex or rare needs, but increasingly they are becoming part of a wider range of other, non-bed-based Tier 4 CAMHS services which can deliver the same or better outcomes. However, inpatient services still play a crucial role in meeting the needs of young people with the most complex or risky mental health difficulties.

In this chapter the clinical pathway into and out of an inpatient unit is described, including the assessment procedure and aims and indications for admission. The work and role of the inpatient unit is outlined, including the types of difficulty presenting for treatment; theories of change; the therapeutic interventions; staff usually available and the evidence for the effectiveness of inpatient treatment, including predictors of a good outcome.

The range of inpatient services

The majority of inpatient units are general purpose, in that they admit young people with a variety of disorders, offering a number of different interventions. Even within general purpose units, some degree of division can occur, for example for different age ranges. Commonly, children's units will take from the age of 5 years up until about 13–14 years, and adolescent units from 13–14 up to 16 or 18 years.

There are also a number of units that provide a more specialist service. Some units treat specific disorders, for example eating disorders, learning disabilities or drug and alcohol problems. Other units offer a specialist intervention or environment, for example forensic units, acute or planned admission units, intensive care units and secure units. Unless otherwise stated, this chapter focuses on the work of a general purpose inpatient unit.

However, it is worth noting that general purpose inpatient units have come under increasing pressure to manage both acute and planned admissions within the same environment. Young people admitted by these different routes often have quite different and mutually exclusive needs. For example, a young person experiencing an acute psychotic episode may need immediate admission and benefit from a safe, containing, low stimulus environment, whereas those with an eating disorder or severe self-harm and suicidality have better outcomes if admission is planned and an active, stimulating and motivating therapeutic programme is provided. It is difficult to meet the different needs of these youngsters in a single environment. Recognition of this has resulted in many general purpose units separating acute from planned admissions, with either completely separate buildings or buildings co-located with some interventions shared.

How many inpatient beds are needed?

In order to estimate how many inpatient beds should be commissioned, ideally we should start with an estimate of the number of young people that have severe and complex mental health needs requiring admission. However, this is a complicated task. There are approximately 12 million children and young people below the age of 18 years in the UK, with approximately 10 per cent (1.2 million) with a diagnosable mental health difficulty (Office for National Statistics, 2004). Community CAMHS (Tier 3) see approximately 250,000 children per year. There are currently approximately 1,130 beds in the UK in 91 inpatient units taking about 2,500 admissions a year (O'Herlihy et al., 2007), This suggests that fewer than 1 per cent of all those in treatment with CAMHS are admitted at any one time. Is this the right proportion?

It is extremely difficult to gauge absolute need for inpatient provision without taking the full range of other CAMHS services into account, including those provided by social care, education and youth justice agencies. In addition, the presence of day units or specialist outpatient and community services will affect the demand on inpatient beds. Defining the purpose of inpatient facilities is also an essential part of quantifying need. It is generally accepted that inpatient facilities provide assessment and management of those young people with severe and/or complex problems that cannot be managed in Tier 3 CAMHS or other community services (Royal College of Psychiatrists, 2007). Specific criteria, however, vary between units, for example around age range, treatment of young people with learning disabilities and the relative priority given to treating emerging personality disorder.

Guidelines from the Royal College of Psychiatrists (2006) suggest a need for 20–40 child and adolescent mental health beds for young people up to their sixteenth birthday per million of general population. In the UK we currently fall short of this, especially when the need for CAMHS beds for 16- and 17-year-olds is taken into account. The distribution of beds also varies considerably across the country with South-East England the only part of the UK to get near to Royal College of Psychiatrists recommendations (O'Herlihy et al., 2007).

Whilst there is a good case to argue that we need more of all types of inpatient facilities, there is a particular lack of emergency access to beds and a lack of intensive support facilities within the NHS (Cotgrove et al., 2007). These gaps should be addressed as a high priority by establishing specialist units to complement rather than replace existing services.

Referral, assessment and aims of admission

Pathways of referral – stepped care approach

In 1995 the Health Advisory Service (HAS) published *Together We Stand* outlining their recommendations for the future of CAMHS. Three main themes came out of this document:

1 recognition of the need for improved cooperation, collaboration and integration between existing services and disciplines;
2 need for the further development of services for older adolescents and young adults;
3 development of a four tier child and adolescent mental health service, with an emphasis on developing the role of a 'primary mental healthcare worker'.

The four tiers described are summarised in more detail in Chapter 1. Inpatient units and other specialist services are located within Tier 4 CAMHS. Non-bed-based services are described in detail elsewhere in this book, but it is important to understand how inpatient units can complement and relate to other specialist services. Coherent care pathways are needed to avoid duplication or gaps in service delivery. This section explores the process and criteria for admission, considering alternatives where appropriate.

Inpatient units generally act as tertiary referral centres, accepting referrals primarily from other specialist services, such as community child and adolescent mental health services.

BOX 3.1   Inpatient assessment procedure

1   Is admission desirable?
2   Are the presenting problems likely to be helped by admission?
3   Is there motivation to change? (Clear aims and objectives can help clarify this.)
4   Are there any suitable alternatives?
5   Could admission cause more harm than benefit?

Assessment procedure

The aim of an assessment is to establish if an admission is desirable and explore what the alternatives are to admission. This simple statement is often complex to address. Box 3.1 summarises the main questions which need to be taken into account.

In order to ascertain whether a young person's difficulties are likely to improve with an admission to an inpatient unit, a full psychiatric and systemic assessment is necessary. This can be done in a number of ways and does not necessarily mean that professionals from the inpatient unit need to gather all this information first-hand. To avoid duplication, much of this information can be gathered from referrers who often know the young person best.

In some cases it is useful to suggest a professionals meeting, where all those who have been involved in the case meet to share information. This can also facilitate consideration of alternatives to a possible admission to an inpatient unit, as well as help plan an admission if this is considered the best option. Whilst information from the referrer and other professionals can be extremely useful and save duplication, it is not a substitute for a direct assessment with the young person and their family. This is needed to clarify with the young person and their family what ideas they have about who or what needs to change, and how they think an inpatient unit may or may not be helpful. Such information is vital in planning possible treatment approaches with the adolescent and their families. It also allows the professionals to start engaging with the adolescent and their family and exploring motivations for change.

There are various aspects to, and different parties involved in, understanding the motivation for the referral to an inpatient unit. It is desirable, but not essential, to have motivation and cooperation from the young person, their family and the referrer. This needs to be based on informed consent and it is important that the young person and usually their family have a clear idea about what is on offer and know something about how the inpatient unit works. In some cases, such as in the treatment of anorexia nervosa, an admission is far more likely to be successful when there is a clear motivation to change on the part of the young person and their family (Ainsworth, 1984; Cotgrove, 2001). For other young people, such as those with psychotic disorders, inpatient treatment may still be indicated without it. Referrer support and cooperation with the treatment package is also desirable, particularly when negotiating admission and follow-up after discharge. Conversely, it may be that the young person and their family have no motivation for change or to receive treatment, and the customer for the service is the referrer or another professional. In such cases admission is only likely to follow if it is supported by legislation such as the Mental Health Act 1983, the Children Act 1989, or by the granting of a Wardship Order. This area is explored further in Chapter 14.

Where possible, clear aims and objectives for admission should be agreed between the young person, their parents or carers, the referrer and the clinical team. These aims can be helpful in clarifying motivation for change, but also to gauge progress during admission. Such aims can range from quite small, quantifiable changes, such as reducing excessive hand washing, to broader aims, such as improving self-esteem. However, even with grander aims it can be helpful to clarify examples of how these might be measured and attempt to monitor improvement by, for example, using a rating scale. The goal-based outcome (GBO) measure developed by the CAMHS Outcome Research Consortium (CORC) is a good example of how using aims can be standardised and provide a measure of outcome (CAMHS Outcome Research Consortium, 2007; Pender et al., 2013). Whatever the aims, even if they are difficult to measure, they need to be realistic, and preferably SMART (specific, measurable, achievable, relevant and timely).

The issue of whether an admission could cause more harm than good is one which clinicians, in their enthusiasm to be helpful can sometimes overlook, but which should always be considered. An admission is less likely to be harmful when it is agreed by the young person, their family, the referrer and the assessing professionals from the inpatient unit, and there are clear SMART aims for that admission. Even in these circumstances there are possible risks, including increased dependence and institutionalisation. More concerning is when a young person is forced into an admission against their will. It can be a major step, particularly for the younger and less mature child, to be removed from their families and other support networks, and even with the best intentions such a step should not be taken lightly. It is possible, on occasions, that this experience could be traumatic and compound problems which already exist. Generally, such a step should only be considered when admission is needed to ensure the young person's safety, where there is evidence of abuse or neglect in the home, and/or there is good evidence that inpatient treatment will improve the youngster's mental health.

Consideration should be given to the location of the initial assessment. Once invited to an inpatient unit, a family will have some degree of expectation that an offer of admission will follow. In some cases, such expectations may be followed by disappointment or a sense of rejection if admission is not offered. It can be helpful then to make a judgement from the information passed on by the referrer and other professionals as to the likelihood that an admission will follow. If it seems likely that alternatives to admission will be recommended, then it may be helpful to carry out the initial assessment at the referrer's base, or in the family home. This can also help give the message that responsibility for the case remains with the referrer at the time of the initial assessment.

The age of the young person, both chronological and developmental, needs to be taken into account as part of the assessment. For example, when deciding between a children's unit or an adolescent unit, a pre-pubertal child with some educational difficulties, even if their chronological age fits the admission criteria for an adolescent unit, may be more appropriate receiving treatment in a specialist children's unit. Working with an age range which overlaps with both children's inpatient services and adult services allows for flexibility in this regard.

With increasing pressure for inpatient units to admit young people in a crisis immediately it may not always be possible to cover all the aspects of an assessment described above. This is especially true with out-of-hours admissions. Whist it is to be welcomed that inpatient services are responsive to young people in crisis, accepting admissions without a thorough assessment can result in many admissions that would better be better managed with non-bed-based services. Such services are described throughout this book.

In addition to providing assessments for the suitability of an admission, inpatient service staff may be asked to provide a second opinion or a consultation to facilitate planning future management. As specialist community-based Tier 4 services are patchy nationwide, inpatient units sometimes provide the main source of expertise in severe and complex mental health issues.

Indications for admission

In UK studies Garralda (1986) and Wolkind and Gent (1987), found criteria for admission included failure of outpatient treatment, difficulties with assessment or diagnosis, family difficulties and the need for 24-hour observation or care. Wrate et al. (1994) in a UK multi-centre prospective study looked at reasons for admission in 276 young people admitted to specialised adolescent psychiatric units. The reasons given are shown in Box 3.2.

Further surveys of criteria for admission to inpatient units have been carried out in the US (Costello et al., 1991; Pottick et al., 1995). These studies generally replicate the UK findings, but also include factors specific to the US, such as the presence of insurance cover (Pottick et al., 1995). Costello et al. (1991) developed a checklist of criteria which had good predictive value when determining whether or not a child needed admission. However, admission rates in the US are much higher than the UK, one study suggesting by approximately five times (Maskey, 1998). Clearly, caution is needed in applying such findings to settings in the UK.

BOX 3.2   Reasons for admission

- provide a detailed psychiatric assessment (51 per cent);
- establish better therapeutic control of a case (36 per cent);
- provide a therapeutic peer group experience (36 per cent);
- obtain improved control over the adolescent's behaviour (26 per cent);
- relieve outpatient colleagues from a treatment failure (20 per cent);
- assess or facilitate future placement needs (19 per cent);
- provide relief to exhausted parents (18 per cent);
- achieve psychological separation between parents and the patient (17 per cent);
- provide an outpatient with schooling otherwise unavailable (9 per cent).

Source: Adapted from Wrate et al. (1994).

Admission criteria in the UK continue to vary between individual inpatient units, but generally now fall into three broad categories (see Cotgrove, 2001; Green, 2002; NICE, 2005).

1 *High risk:* admission may be indicated when there are high levels of risk to the child or young person, secondary to suicidal thoughts or behaviours or self-neglect, and beyond the capacity of the family and community-based services to manage. Admission should be expected to reduce this risk.
2 *Intensive treatment:* when the intensity of treatment needed is not available from other services. This is commonly the case when a disorder is associated with other psychosocial difficulties, and/or co-morbid disorder resulting in difficulties pervading all aspects of the child/young person's life.
3 *Intensive assessment:* an inpatient unit can offer 24-hours-a-day assessment and supervision by a multidisciplinary team to gather information to guide further management. This may involve observing the child or young person's behaviour and their interaction with others, observing the effects of a specific intervention, such as the use of medication, or allowing time for a range of investigations to be carried out, such as cognitive assessments or physical investigations. The admission can also allow for the assessment of the young person's difficulties out of the context of their home or school. For example, a young person may appear severely depressed in the context of a problematic home environment or associated with bullying at school, but their mood may lift significantly when admitted. This information can be helpful in guiding future management whether or not further inpatient treatment is indicated. Inpatient assessment may also aid diagnosis. Young people with features of an emerging personality disorder, for example, may present with variable mood, including depression. Evidence of such co-morbid disorders can help guide future management. It should be noted, however, that much of this information may be obtainable whilst the young person remains in the community, and admission should never be seen as an alternative to a good community assessment.

Contraindications or risks of admission

It is important when considering an admission that the potential benefits are balanced against potential harm. There is a range of reasons why inpatient treatment may not be appropriate:

a There may be concerns about admitting a particularly vulnerable young person into an environment where there are high levels of disturbance potentially compounding their distress.
b A vulnerable young person admitted to an environment with high levels of self-harm or acting out behaviours is at risk of acquiring additional dysfunctional behaviours or coping strategies, even where a skilled and experienced staff team openly address such difficulties.

c   If protracted, an admission runs the risk of 'institutionalising' the young person, including loss of support from their community network, and detrimental effects on family life (Green & Jones, 1998).

d   Inpatient treatments are expensive (e.g. Green et al., 2001).

For these reasons inpatient admission is often considered a last resort.

Aims of admission

There are increasing numbers of inpatient services accepting emergency admissions of young people in crisis. For many of these the immediate risk or crisis will have reduced with a day or a few days. It is important that when the crisis has subsided discharge is facilitated as soon as possible with a suitable package of support in the community. Even those with high risk may still be better managed in the community with appropriate support as the risks of inpatient admission may outweigh the risks of discharge in some cases. What follows largely applies to those that need longer-term inpatient treatment due to the complexity and severity of their needs or ongoing high levels of risk that can be reduced by inpatient treatment.

Most admissions to Tier 4 inpatient settings happen 'informally'. This means either that the child or young person has agreed to come into hospital and accept help with their mental health problems or their parent has consented. This is important since commitment to receiving help is linked to better outcomes for this group. On other occasions, where the young person does not recognise or agree that they require hospital admission, and the risks are such they cannot remain at home, the Mental Health Act 1983 may be used to provide compulsion and admit young people to hospital against their wishes.

Once it is established that an admission is indicated, there are a number of ways in which an admission to an inpatient unit may be helpful. The most obvious of these is to help with the difficulties which have been identified during the assessment procedure. These can include problems raised by the young person and their family, such as to reduce self-harming behaviour or to improve relationships within the family, or may be defined by professionals, for example, to treat a psychotic illness.

There are other aims or benefits from an admission which can be achieved that may not be identified during the assessment. First, an admission may facilitate positive changes in a young person's lifestyle. For example, supportive feedback can result in improvements in self-care. Admission to an inpatient unit may be the first significant period the youngster has spent away from home; this then can be an opportunity for them to increase their sense of self-responsibility, their feelings of independence and reduce dependency on their parents or carers.

Second, an inpatient admission can provide an opportunity for a positive peer group experience, where previously a young person may have felt isolated or been bullied by their peers. This positive experience can improve their ability to make friends and form relationships with others, which, along with other achievements during an inpatient's stay, can improve the young person's self-esteem and feelings of self-worth.

TABLE 3.1   Range of psychiatric disorders treated in a general purpose adolescent unit

Disorder (ICD-10)	%
Psychotic disorder F20-29	12
Mood disorder (including bipolar) F30-39	28
Neurotic disorder F40-49	12
Eating disorder F50-59	18
Emerging emotionally unstable personality disorder F60-69	9
Developmental disorder F80-89	6
Behavioural and emotional disorder F90-99	13

Source: Van Niekerk and Cotgrove (2012).

Finally, an aim for any admission should be to reduce the risk of, or severity of, long-term psychopathology. An intensive inpatient experience has the potential to impact significantly on the personality development of a young person. This can then impact on the trajectory the young person may embark on through life, shifting it from one of repeated recourse to psychiatric or psychological services, to one where the individual acquires the personal resources to be more effective in resolving future difficulties, enabling them to find personal fulfilment and happiness in life.

Range of disorders commonly treated in inpatient units

Inpatient units treat young people with a range of psychiatric conditions. Table 3.1 shows the diagnostic breakdown of the primary International Classification of Diseases (ICD)-10 axis 1 diagnoses made in a general purpose adolescent unit averaged over a 5-year period, 2006–2011 (Van Niekerk & Cotgrove, 2012). Whilst there remains variation between units, these figures are fairly typical for a general purpose service (see O'Herlihy et al., 2003).

ICD-10 diagnoses can help give a picture of the range of difficulties presenting to an inpatient unit, but only from one perspective. For example, if categorising according to behaviours such as self-harm and suicidal behaviour, almost 40 per cent of admissions show these behaviours.

Theories and models of change

Inpatient units increasingly work towards discharging young people as quickly as it is safe to do so. Aims for admission are often, and rightly, focused on what needs to change to allow the young person to return home. However, those units that have the potential to work with young people for a sustained period can provide an experience for a young person which has the potential to have a profound effect on their personality development. The next section on 'therapeutic interventions' outlines the range of treatments commonly used in an inpatient unit. First, however, in this section a theoretical model based on attachment theory is used to describe how a non-specific, intense and extensive therapeutic experience for a young person in an inpatient unit could positively change the trajectory of their personality development, thus reducing the risk of severe life long psychopathology. This model is not intended to represent the 'truth' about what happens in adolescent units, but hopefully a helpful way to consider the issues.

Attachment theory

Attachment theory emphasises the importance and biological function of intimate relationships between individuals, the central role of caregivers on a child's development, and the persistence of attachment styles throughout life. For the development of a secure attachment a child needs to be sure that should he encounter any frightening or adverse situations, his parents will respond in a predictable and helpful way. When this occurs the child is able to use the attachment figure as a secure base from which to explore the world and play returning for comfort should the need arise (Bowlby, 1969).

As the child develops he becomes able to internalise and generalise the pattern of attachment. When a child's care is disrupted by inconsistent, abusive or invalidating parenting a positive secure attachment style is unlikely to develop. Instead the child is likely to become ambivalent to the caregivers, seeking but then rejecting comfort. This may have a profound effect on their ability to form relationships throughout their life. Ambivalent attachment patterns have been shown to be strongly associated with poor personality development and the acquisition of personality difficulties such as those associated with borderline personality disorder (Patrick et al., 1994). Conversely, an experience of consistent, sensitive and responsive parenting in childhood will improve the individual's resilience to adversity.

Whilst there are no studies classifying the attachment patterns of young people admitted to inpatient units, it is clear that many have suffered extremes of adversity in terms of neglect and abuse in childhood and display many of the features of borderline personality functioning. It is therefore essential that staff understand attachment theory and how insecure or unstable attachments can manifest. Negotiating a contract for admission with clear aims and objectives can provide material for the content of the therapeutic work carried out during an admission. However, the inpatient unit also has the opportunity to provide a safe, caring and containing environment, in which this work can be carried out. For some the experience of consistent and responsive care giving as provided by the staff group may be new, and over a period of time could be internalised. Such an internalised 'secure base' can give the adolescent a new repertoire for relating to people in a positive way, which may then have positive implications for other aspects of their personality functioning such as self-esteem. Thus, overall there is the potential, through a change in internalised attachment constructs, to profoundly affect the trajectory of the young person's personality development.

Should this be the role of an inpatient unit? For many young people with attachment difficulties it is their home environment that should provide the consistent, containing and responsive care that the young person needs. However, for a small proportion of young people with attachment difficulties associated with other severe and complex mental health needs, and where all other options have been exhausted, there may be no safe or effective alternatives to inpatient admission.

Therapeutic interventions and philosophies

Attachment theory has been used as an example to illustrate how a consistent approach to caring for adolescents in an inpatient setting can have a positive impact on their personality development, particularly for those who have had inadequate or abusive caregiving early in life. Other developmental models can be used to justify the value of such an approach, including psychoanalytic or cognitive psychological models.

Whilst a particular theory, model or philosophy may underpin the thinking or therapeutic structure of an inpatient unit, the day to day treatments involved tend to be varied and multiple to reflect the individual needs of young people with a wide range of disorders. Hence, in practice, the therapeutic milieu of an average general purpose inpatient unit tends to be eclectic. Programmes are designed to treat specific disorders and alleviate symptomatic disturbance, as well as promoting self-esteem, consolidating a stable sense of identity, improving confidence to manage independent living and the formation of realistic vocational goals. Various National Institute for Health and Care Excellence (NICE) guidelines summarise the evidence available to guide clinicians in the treatments they offer for specific disorders.

The range of therapeutic interventions used in a typical inpatient unit are summarised in Box 3.3.

BOX 3.3   Therapeutic interventions used in inpatient units

Therapeutic milieu:
- Safe, containing and responsive environment, i.e. 'secure base'.

Specific therapies:
- Group work including:
    - group psychotherapy;
    - art and drama therapy;
    - outward bound activities;
    - social skills;
    - coping strategies.

Family therapy:
- Individual work including:
    - cognitive and behaviour therapy;
    - dialectical behaviour therapy;
    - psychodynamic therapy;
    - daily living skills.

Psychopharmacology

The therapeutic milieu

Generally, inpatient units have a core of communal activities which involve most or all of the young people. This usually includes regular community meetings, when staff and young people can discuss day-to-day practical issues arising from the young people living together. Sometimes such meetings also include the discussion of individual emotional difficulties, or problems the young people may have in their relationships with each other. Schooling or other educational activities also often form part of the core life of an inpatient unit, and in some units most of the 'working day' will be taken up in educational activities.

Beyond these core activities, the ratio of communal therapeutic activity to specific individual therapy is quite variable. Historically, many inpatient units drew on therapeutic community principles whereby little or no specific individual work took place. Whilst this mode of working is no longer viable for the general purpose adolescent unit which has to treat a wide range of disorders using evidence-based interventions, some principles are still used. Therapeutic programmes can be designed to try and make all the activities throughout the day in some way therapeutic. This model of working can have some significant advantages in terms of using the peer group to facilitate positive change, and to encourage the taking on of responsibilities. Practical activities such as planning, shopping for and cooking meals together can have a range of benefits, such as developing cooperative and relationship skills, improving basic living skills as well as benefiting self-esteem by providing a meal which others will eat and compliment.

Other group activities can include developing coping strategies, particularly for young people who self-harm, group psychotherapy, creative therapies, such as art and drama, and outward bound activity. However, group work in an inpatient or day patient setting can have the added power of working with a group of young people who are also spending a great deal of the rest of their day to day lives together. This can enable them to work on relationship skills by looking at their relationships with each other in an intensity that would not normally be available in outpatient group work. Creative therapies such as art and drama therapy and outward bound activities can provide an opportunity for adolescents to work on their emotional difficulties as well as relationship issues in ways that do not rely as heavily as some on verbal communication skills. For example, a young person may be able to express feelings of hopelessness and despair in a painting, in a way they could never express verbally. Similarly, outward bound activities sometimes allow young people to excel in their physical abilities or cooperative group abilities when otherwise they may see themselves as low achievers.

Whilst such a 'therapeutic milieu' of group activities can have significant benefits for many young people, occasionally it can be in an individual's best interest not to take part in some aspects of the programme. The overall effect of participating in the group activities can be quite stimulating and arousing, and for some, such as those in an acute psychotic episode, it is better to participate in lower stimulus activities. Even with such cases, the structure of a clear timetable for the day can have an important containing effect.

Individual work

The amount of individual therapy carried out within an inpatient unit is variable. Apart from the intensity with which psychological therapies may be used, their benefits are much the same in an inpatient as outpatient setting. Some units develop specific individual therapeutic programmes, which may include individual cognitive or behaviour therapy, individual psychodynamic psychotherapy and individual task setting. Specific individual therapies include exposure and response prevention programmes for the treatment of obsessive–compulsive symptoms, behavioural programmes to help with agoraphobia, or some supportive counselling to discuss in private some particularly traumatic or abusive experiences. In order to maintain links with community services and facilitate rapid discharge, it can sometime be useful to use a community CAMHS therapist for individual work.

Family work

Family work is generally considered an essential part of the work of most adolescent units for those that have longer stays. In an inpatient setting work carried out with the family will often parallel that which is provided in an outpatient setting; however, there are some additional benefits. Family work allows there to be a formal, regular exchange of views regarding the young person's progress. The parents can find out about their child's progress and any difficulties at the unit and the family workers have an opportunity to gain information about how the young person is progressing in their parents' eyes, for example when they are home on weekend leave. This information can be useful both in direct therapeutic work with the family and also to guide further work within the inpatient unit.

Psychopharmacology

The place for the use of psychopharmacology in inpatient units is well recognised. As with other therapeutic interventions NICE guidelines provide recommendations on the role of specific medications for each of the main disorders. For some disorders there are specific guidelines for children and young people, whilst for others we extrapolate from adult guidance. Occasionally admission to an inpatient unit can enable assessment and containment of quite worrying symptomatology without recourse to medication in the first instance. This can be particularly helpful when assessing adolescents presenting with a depressive disorder, where the evidence for the efficacy of medication is weak and when admission may result in a resolution of many of the symptoms suggesting a large environmental component to that individual's difficulties, or evidence of emotional dysregulation, rather than a pervasive depressive disorder, emerges.

Staffing

Multidisciplinary teams will contain representatives from some or all of the following professions: psychiatrists, mental health or children's nurses, social workers, psychologists and teachers. There will also be administrative and secretarial staff. Other specialist input may be provided by psychotherapists, creative therapists such as art, drama or music therapists, occupational therapists and research and academic staff. Each of these disciplines may also have trainees passing through the unit for limited periods. In addition, most units will employ unqualified staff, such as clinical support workers, or psychology graduates wishing to gain clinical experience.

All adolescent units will have their own unique mix of the above staff, both in proportions and in absolute numbers. The Royal College of Psychiatrists (2006) have produced guidelines for recommended minimum staffing levels. Most adolescent units will have enough nursing staff to provide care and therapeutic input 24 hours a day. This will inevitably result in nurses out numbering most other disciplines, and perhaps being seen, and seeing themselves, as the core of the unit. Although smaller in numbers, psychiatrists and teachers are commonly the other key professionals. Whilst the doctors and nurses share some medical training and experience, a teacher's professional background is quite separate. In terms of their roles, it generally falls upon the nursing staff to provide day-to-day care and containment for the children or young people, as well as, to a greater or lesser extent, to provide specific therapeutic activities. Psychiatrists tend to take on the role of assessing young people with more complex mental health problems, including mental state assessments. They may also take on a leadership role, with clinical responsibility for the care of specific young people resting with a consultant psychiatrist. However, leadership is sometimes shared by senior professionals of different disciplines.

The roles of teachers and the importance of schooling vary quite considerably between adolescent units. In some units the schooling may be set up quite separately by a team of teachers who are solely involved in the educational side of the service. In other units, schooling takes on a smaller role and the teachers are involved in a range of activities around the unit.

Social workers can have a particular role in liaising with local authorities over accommodation issues for 'looked after' young people and should have expertise in child protection matters. Psychologists can provide psychometric assessments and often have particular therapeutic skills, such as in cognitive behaviour therapy or cognitive analytic therapy. The primary role of other staff such as psychotherapists, art and drama therapists, administrative and secretarial staff is clearly suggested by their professional title.

The way the rest of the work, including assessments, second opinions, general milieu therapy and specific therapies, such as individual, group and family therapy is allocated, depends partly on the philosophy of the unit and partly on the skills of the individuals involved. In some units this work may be divided up irrespective of profession or discipline, whereas in others professions such as psychiatrists, psychologists and nurses may take the lead in carrying out assessments and specific therapies.

A particular danger can be to give too much of the responsibility for the general milieu therapy to the untrained or least skilled members of staff without adequate supervision. Such staff can sometimes befriend young people, becoming the preferred therapist, but as the least skilled and experienced there is a risk of them transgressing boundaries. It is therefore vital that such staff are given training and a high level of supervision as part of their induction and during their employment.

Evidence of effectiveness

The research evidence for the efficacy of inpatient treatment is limited for most, if not all, psychiatric disorders across the age range. A systematic review of the literature revealed only one randomised controlled trial (RCT) specifically looking at admission as a treatment modality for children and young people, but there are a range of other studies using other research methodologies.

Henggeler et al. (1999) conducted an RCT in the US comparing home-based multisystemic therapy (MST) with brief (1–2 week) inpatient psychiatric hospitalisation. MST offers a range of therapeutic interventions designed to impact on multiple determinants of the youngster's key problems arising from the individual, family, peers, school and community. It is notable that 44 per cent of the home-based treatment sample also received hospitalisation. Hospitalisation was more effective in improving young people's self-esteem. MST was more effective in decreasing the young people's externalising (behavioural) symptoms.

A small number of controlled trials comparing inpatient treatment with outpatient treatment have been carried out in the US. Flomenhaft (1974) and Winsberg et al. (1980) just looked at young people with antisocial behaviour or externalising disorder. Rothery et al. (1995) reviewed outcomes according to a set of 16 predetermined treatment goals and diagnosis in a multi-centre study of 320 consecutive admissions to four specialist adolescent units in the UK. Overall the outcomes for inpatient treatment were positive.

Sheerin et al. (1999), studied a sample of 29 consecutive admissions (results from 26 reported) to a psychiatric inpatient unit for children aged 3 to 13 years (mean age 8.6 years) in Scotland. At 3-month and 15-month post-discharge follow-up they found a significant reduction in symptoms.

Green et al. (2001), in an English study, looked at 55 consecutive admissions of children and adolescents aged 6 to 17 years (mean age 11.4 years) to two inpatient units from late 1995 to 1997. Measures using the Children's Global Assessment Scale (CGAS) (Shaffer et al., 1983) and the Health of the Nation Outcome Scale (Child and Adolescent Mental Health) (HoNOSCA) (Gowers et al. 1999) showed no significant changes between referral and admission (waiting list control). Median waiting list time was 3 months. Significant health gain was found on most measures by discharge and sustained at follow-up.

Jacobs et al. (2004) have repeated the Green et al. (2001) study on a larger scale ($n = 155$). The sample consisted of sequential admissions of children and adolescents aged 3 to 17 years (mean age 13.9 years) to eight UK inpatient units (four child, four adolescent) between January 2001 and April 2002. A range of measures were used to monitor symptom change and health gain before admission, during admission and one year following discharge. Significant improvements were found in global functioning, psychopathology and 'cardinal problem' measures at discharge, which were maintained at one year follow-up. This compared with a much smaller (although still significant) improvement whilst on the waiting list.

Gowers et al. (2000) used the HoNOSCA, a crude outcome measure rated by the treating clinician, on 35 consecutive admissions to an adolescent unit in England. This showed significant reductions in HoNOSCA scores between admission and discharge of 18.0 to 9.3 respectively in clinician rated scores ($p < 0.001$) and 18.3 to 12.6 respectively in user rated scores ($p < 0.001$). Similar positive findings were made in a subsequent study with larger numbers (137 consecutive admissions) by van Niekerk and Cotgrove (2012).

Predictors of outcome

Pfeiffer and Strzelecki (1990) carried out a literature search to look for publications on outcome and follow-up investigations of residential and inpatient psychiatric hospitalisations between 1975 and 1990. Thirty-four studies were identified. When analysing the findings weightings were applied that reflected sample size. They found a positive relationship between good outcome and the following factors:

- specific characteristics of treatments (e.g. completion of treatment programme, planned discharge and therapeutic alliance);
- the use of after care;
- level of family functioning and involvement with treatment;
- length of stay (longer);
- higher intelligence.

Some symptom areas were found to be associated with poorer outcomes, such as:

- presence of psychotic symptoms;
- bizarre symptoms;
- antisocial behaviours;
- under-socialised aggressive conduct disorder.

Kutash and Rivera (1996) carried out a systematic review of subsequent studies using a similar methodology, finding additional support for Pfeiffer and Strzelecki's conclusions and in particular underscoring the benefit of family participation.

More recent studies have confirmed and clarified the following factors as predictors of outcome: length of stay (Sheerin et al., 1999; Green et al., 2001; Jacobs et al., 2004); therapeutic alliance between the child and their family with the inpatient team, and family participation in the therapeutic process (Green et al., 2001; Jacobs et al., 2004); pre-admission family functioning (King et al., 1997; Green et al., 2001); and severity of depressive symptoms (King et al., 1997).

Van Niekerk and Cotgrove (2012) looked at outcomes in consecutive admissions to an adolescent unit, as measured by HoNOSCA, over a 5-year period. Average HoNOSCA scores dropped from 19 to 10.6 during admission. Outcome scores correlated with diagnosis, those with psychotic disorders and mood disorders improving by 53 per cent, neurotic disorders and behavioural and emotional disorders by 35 per cent, developmental disorders by 35 per cent, eating disorders by 35 per cent and those with emerging personality disorders by 25 per cent.

For some young people, particularly those at high risk of self-harm or neglect, or needing intensive assessment and/or treatment, there is often no alternative to inpatient admission. In summary, there are a number of studies suggesting that young people with a range of mental health disorders have good outcomes from a period of admission. Clinical factors which appear to predict outcome, include: specific characteristics of treatments (e.g. completion of treatment programme, planned discharge and therapeutic alliance), the use of after care, the level of family functioning pre-admission, the level of family involvement with treatment, length of stay (longer), and higher intelligence. Also those with psychosis and mood disorders appear to do better than those with emerging borderline personality disorder. Little is known about the impact of service and treatment variables within the inpatient setting.

Standards of care

Over the last decade the Quality Network for Inpatient CAMHS (QNIC) (Royal College of Psychiatrists, 2011) has developed a range of standards for inpatient units to aspired to, and be measured against. There are seven main areas that QNIC standards cover:

1   Environment and Facilities;
2   Staffing and Training;
3   Access, Admission and Discharge;
4   Care and Treatment;
5   Information, Consent and Confidentiality;
6   Young People's Rights and Safeguarding;
7   Clinical Governance.

Inpatient units are able to self-assess where they are up to in each of the standards and there are annual peer reviews where professionals from the network visit units and assess adherence to the standards. One great advantage to this system over other methods of regulation and compliance is it allows for a degree of peer support and information sharing. For more details please see Chapter 13 on quality standards.

Commissioning

Inpatient units have historically been commissioned in a variety of different ways. The Carter Review of Commissioning Arrangements for Specialist Services (Department of Health, 2006) recommended that Tier 4 CAMHS be commissioned by specialist commissioning teams. This view has been reiterated in the NHS Specialised Services National Definition Set (NHS, 2010). However, this recommendation has not yet been fully implemented across the country. With the disbanding of PCTs and the introduction of Local Area Teams (LATs) and Clinical Commissioning Groups (CCGs), it is not clear at the time of writing who will pick up commissioning for the full range of Tier 4 services. However, it is looking increasingly clear that inpatient Tier 4 services will be commissioned by NHS England. A National Service Specification has been developed which will be used as a template for commissioners.

There is currently no consistent approach to the currency used for commissioning. Many services are block contracted for the number of beds provided, whilst others are funded according to activity. This variation occurs both within NHS provided services and the independent sector. Please see Chapter 12 for further details of commissioning in Tier 4 CAMHS.

Conclusions

The inpatient unit has evolved considerably over recent decades. Twenty to thirty years ago they were often led by charismatic leaders with idiosyncratic operational policies. With little evidence base to guide them, therapeutic practice was determined by the varied experience of the staff, but often focusing on long term therapeutic interventions for those with complex needs, at the expense of those with serious mental illness such as psychosis.

Throughout their existence some have questioned the value of inpatient services, in particular people that believed that a combination of prevention and intensive non-bed-based interventions could meet all young people's needs. Now, few would question the need to have some inpatient services, but beds are seen as part of a range of services to meet the needs of those young people with complex and severe difficulties. It is also increasingly recognised that inpatient services are needed for young people in crisis, as well as those needing longer-term planned treatments. It is difficult to address both these sets of needs in a single environment, so many units are now separating services for acute admissions from planned admissions.

The next decade is likely to see a further development in specialist non-bed-based services to work alongside and in conjunction with inpatient units. There is further work needed in many areas to establish robust gate-keeping services to prevent unnecessary admissions and make the most effective use of the beds we have. In addition, long-standing gaps in provision between social care and health, particularly for those young people experiencing distress in conjunction with family breakdown, need to be addressed to prevent inappropriate referrals for admission.

References

Ainsworth, P. (1984) The first 100 admissions to a regional general purpose adolescent unit. *Journal of Adolescence* 7, 337–348.

Bowlby, J. (1969) *Attachment and Loss*. London: Hogarth Press.

CAMHS Outcome Research Consortium (2007) *Goal-based Outcome Measure*. www.corc.uk.net

Costello, A., Dulcan, M. & Kalas, R. (1991) A checklist of hospitalisation criteria for use with children. *Hospital & Community Psychiatry*, 42, 823–828.

Cotgrove, A. (2001) The adolescent unit. In S. Gowers (Ed.) *Adolescent Psychiatry in Clinical Practice* (pp. 321–345). London: Arnold.

Cotgrove, A., McLoughlin, R., O'Herlihy, A., & Lelliottt, P. (2007) The ability of adolescent units to accept emergency admissions: changes in England and Wales between 2000 and 2005. *Psychiatric Bulletin*, 31(12), 457–459.

Department of Health (2006) *Review of Commissioning Arrangements for Specialised Services* (The Carter Review). London: Department of Health.

Flomenhaft, K. (1974) Outcome of treatment for adolescents. *Adolescents*, 9, 57–66.

Garralda, E. (1986) In-patient treatment of children: a psychiatric perspective. In G. Edwards (Ed.) *Current issues in Clinical Psychology*, Vol. 4. New York: Plenum Press.

Gowers, S. G., Harrington, R. C., Whitton, A., et al. (1999) Brief scale for measuring the outcomes of emotional and behavioural disorders in children: Health of the Nation Outcome Scales for Children and Adolescents (HoNOSCA). *British Journal of Psychiatry*, 174, 413–416.

Gowers, S., Bailey-Rogers, S., Shone, A. & Levine, W. (2000) The Health of the Nation Outcome Scales for Child and Adolescent Mental Health (HoNOSCA). *Child Psychology and Psychiatry Review*, 5(2), 50–56.

Green, J. (2002) Provision of intensive treatment: in-patient units, day units and intensive outreach. In M. Rutter and E. Taylor (Eds) *Child and Adolescent Psychiatry*, (pp. 1038–1050). London: Blackwell.

Green, J. & Jones, D. (1998) Unwanted effects of in-patient treatment: anticipation, prevention, repair. In J. M. Green and B. W. Jacobs (Eds) *In-patient Child Psychiatry. Modern Practice, Research and the Future* (pp. 212–220). London: Routledge.

Green, J., Kroll, L., Imrie, D., Frances, F., Begum, K., Harrison, L. & Anson, R. (2001) Health gain and outcome predictors during in-patient and related day treatment in child and adolescent psychiatry. *Journal of American Academy of Child and Adolescent Psychiatry*, 40(3), 325–332.

Health Advisory Service (1995) *Together We Stand*. London: HMSO.

Henggeler, S. W., Rowland, M. D., Randall, J., Ward, D. M., Pickrel, S. G., Cunningham, P. B., Miller, S., Edwards, J., Zealberg, J. J., Hand, L. E. & Santos, A. B. (1999) Home-based multisystemic therapy as an alternative to the hospitalisation of youths in psychiatric crisis: clinical outcomes. *Journal of American Academy of Child and Adolescent Psychiatry*, 38(11), 1331–1339.

Jacobs, B., Green, J., Beecham, J., Kroll, L., et al. (2004) *Children and Young Persons Inpatient Evaluation (CHYPIE): A Prospective Outcome Study of Inpatient Child and Adolescent Psychiatry in England*. Presented at the Royal College of Psychiatrists Faculty of Child and Adolescent Psychiatry Annual Residential Conference.

King, C., Hovey, J., Brand, E. & Ghaziuddin, N. (1997) Prediction of positive outcomes for adolescent psychiatric in-patients. *Journal of American Academy of Child and Adolescent Psychiatry*. 36(10), 1434–1442.

Kutash, K. & Rivera, V. (1996) *What Works in Children's Mental Health Services: Uncovering Answers to Critical Questions*. Baltimore, MD: Paul H Brooks.

Maskey, S. (1998) The Process of Admission. In J. M. Green and B. W. Jacobs (Eds) *In-patient Child Psychiatry: Modern Practice Research and the Future* (pp. 39–50). London: Routledge.

NHS (2010) Specialised Services National Definition Set. http://www.specialisedservices.nhs.uk/info/specialised-services-national-definitions

NIHCE 2005, *Depression in Children and Young People*. London: NIHCE.

Office for National Statistics (2004) *Annual Report and Accounts*. London: TSO.

O'Herlihy, A., Worrall, A., Lelliott, P., Jaffa, T., Hill, P. & Banerjee, S. (2003) Distribution and characteristics of in-patient child and adolescent mental health services in England and Wales. *British Journal of Psychiatry*, 183, 547–551.

O'Herlihy, A., Lelliott, P., Bannister, D., Cotgrove, A., Farr, H., & Tullock, S. (2007) Provision of child and adolescent mental health inpatient services in England between 1999 and 2006. *Psychiatric Bulletin*, 31(12), 454–456.

O'Herlihy, A., Worrall, A., Lelliott, P., Jaffa, T., Mears, A., Banerjee, S. & Hill, P. (in press) Characteristics of the residents of in-patient child and adolescent mental health services in England and Wales.

Patrick, M., Hobson, R. P. & Castle, D. (1994) Personality disorder and mental representation, *Journal of Development and Psychopathology*, 6, 375–388.

Pender, F., Tinwell, C., Marsh, E. & Cowell, V. (2013). Evaluating the use of goal-based outcomes as a single patient rated outcome measure across CWP CAMHS: a pilot study. *The Child and Family Clinical Psychology Review*. 1(1), 29–40.

Pfeiffer, S. & Strzelecki, S. (1990) In-patient psychiatric treatment of children and adolescents: a review of outcome studies. *Journal of the American Academy of Child and Adolescent Psychiatry*, 29, 847–853.

Pottick, K., Hansell, S., Gutterman, E. & Raskin White, H. (1995) Factors associated with in-patient and out-patient treatment for children and adolescents with serious mental illness. *Journal of the American Academy of Child and Adolescent Psychiatry*, 34, 425–433.

Royal College of Psychiatrists (2006). *Building and Sustaining Specialist CAMHS*. Council Report 137. London: RCP.

Royal College of Psychiatrists (2007) *The Costs, Outcome and Satisfaction for Inpatient Child and Adolescent Psychiatric Services (COSI-CPAS) Study: Report for the National Co-ordinating Centre for NHS Service Delivery and Organisation (R+D)*. London: NCCSDO.

Royal College of Psychiatrists (2011) *Quality Network for Inpatient CAMHS Service Standards*, 6th Edition. London: RCP.

Rothery, D., Wrate, R., McCabe, R., Aspin, J. & Bryce, G. (1995) Treatment goal-planning outcome findings of a British Prospective multi-centre study of adolescent in-patient units. *Eur Child Adolescent Psychiatry*, 4, 209–220.

Shaffer, D., Gould, M. & Brasic, J. (1983) A children's global assessment scale (CGAS). *Archives of General Psychiatry*, 40, 1228–1231.

Sheerin, T., Maguire, R. & Robinson, J. (1999) A 15 month follow-up study of children admitted to a child psychiatric in-patient unit. *Irish Journal of Psychological Medicine*, 16(3), 97–103.

Van Niekerk L. & Cotgrove, A. (2012) Predictors of outcome in a general purpose adolescent unit: 5 year consecutive case review. Presentation at the Royal College of Psychiatrists Child and Adolescent Faculty Annual Meeting.

Winsberg, B., Bailer, I., Kupietz, S., Botti, E. & Balka, E. (1980) Home versus hospital care for children with behaviour disorders. *Archives of General Psychiatry*, 37, 413–418.

Wolkind, S. and Gent, M. (1987) Children's psychiatric in-patient units: present functions and future directions. Special Issue: Residential Provision. *Maladjustment and Therapeutic Education*, 5, 54–56.

Wrate, R., Rothery, D., McCabe, R., Asprin, J. & Bryce, G. (1994) A prospective multi-centre study of admissions to adolescent in-patient units. *Journal of Adolescence*, 17, 221–237.

4

DAY SERVICES

Anne Worrall-Davies

Key points

- Day care packages typically comprise targeted, five day-a-week interventions offering multi-modal 'bundles' of individual, family and psychopharmacological interventions alongside intensive family therapy and parenting work.
- The evidence for the clinical effectiveness of day services is mixed and much dates back to when day services were generic. It is therefore difficult to extrapolate findings to the current system, or indeed to extrapolate to day service in other countries, as day programmes in North America, the UK and Australasia are vastly different.
- There are no randomised trials comparing day services with inpatient care or other services for children and young people.
- Compared to inpatient and outpatient CAMHS, day services can work round young people's school or college timetables, can offer family appointments early or late in the day and can therefore more easily tailor interventions to individual young people's needs.
- The opportunities for completeness and intensity of day service treatment and observation may be limited. The child may struggle to adapt to being in different environments and in some areas the daily trip to and from the day programme may be long and tiring.

Introduction

Day services in CAMHS have been popular since the 1940s, especially in North America. They have evolved with a bewildering array of ethos and treatment models and this has meant that comparative studies of effectiveness are often meaningless. In the last decade, however, the increasing use of alternatives to inpatient care in CAMHS has focused the role of day services, many of which in the UK at least are linked to inpatient units.

This chapter will look at the types of programmes currently offered by CAMHS day programmes, some of the staffing and ethos issues, will review the evidence for their effectiveness, and briefly discuss issues for the future.

In the UK, most inpatient units offer a day programme, but half of UK day services are stand-alone services (Green & Jacobs 1998; O'Herlihy et al. 2003). This is the case in most other European countries where geography such as large rural areas make it impossible to always link day programmes to inpatient facilities (Ellilä et al. 2005).

Functions of day services

Despite the range of styles mentioned earlier, day services may be grouped by their main function (Green & Worrall-Davies 2008; McDougall et al. 2008):

- Step-up, step-down function: support and transition to/from community CAMHS after/before an inpatient admission.
- Harm reduction: assessment and treatment of disruptive, delinquent or offending behaviours.
- Neuro-developmental assessment and treatment: specialist programmes of care for younger children with autism, ADHD, speech and language disorders or neuropsychiatric conditions.
- Intensive family work: five-day-a-week interventions with whole families.
- Targeted care packages for specific problems, e.g. eating disorders or psychosis.

These functions can be achieved through:

- intensive, targeted five day-a-week treatment packages for children and their families;
- multi-modal treatment strategies with a combination of individual, family and psychopharmacological interventions;
- intensive family therapy and parenting work.

Examples of day services are given in Boxes 4.1, 4.2 and 4.3.

Advantages and disadvantages of CAMHS day services

There are several advantages and disadvantages to day services and it is important to consider them when thinking about intervention.

Advantages

- The flexibility of care that can be provided. Compared to outpatient CAMHS, day services can work round young people's school or college timetables, can offer family appointments early or late in the day more easily, and can individually tailor interventions to young people's needs.
- Management of younger children. Concerns about admitting very young children to inpatient units, particularly those far from their homes, and the dearth of children's CAMHS beds in many countries mean that the option of working intensively with

---

BOX 4.1 Example of a 'partial hospitalisation' programme

The Adolescent Partial Hospitalization Program is an after-school day hospital program targeting adolescents ages 12 through 18. This program offers a complete psychiatric and psychosocial evaluation, occupational therapy assessment, family therapy, nursing support and, if necessary, pharmacotherapy. The patients participate in a variety of groups, including occupational therapy, problem solving, and behavioral psychotherapy. Each adolescent has an individual therapist. Family members are also involved in treatment through weekly family therapy meetings. Socialization and recreation therapies round out the treatment.

Source: http://www.hopkinsmedicine.org/psychiatry/

BOX 4.2 Example of a 'step-up step-down' eating disorders programme

The Eating Disorder Day Programme is a five day-a-week step-up step-down service supporting young people with eating disorders. It is a more intensive option than the CAMHS outreach service but prevents or shortens inpatient stays. Meals are all supported from breakfast to tea in the programme and a range of structured activities, therapeutic groups and formal education are offered.

Source: http://www.WHAT IS WEBSITEcamhs.org.uk/

BOX 4.3 Example of a day programme for young people with severe mental illness

The Adolescent Day Treatment Program (ADTP) supports adolescents who are experiencing severe psychiatric difficulties such as psychotic, mood and anxiety disorders, and who are also struggling with their academic, family, and social functioning. It provides a viable treatment alternative for young people who do not require hospitalization, but who need intensive, structured mental health programming, as well as educational programming when the school system cannot meet their needs. A broad range of recovery oriented treatment and support is offered through a safe and structured environment.

Source: http://www.fraserhealth.ca

---

young children is often limited. Outreach and day programmes are crucial for providing 24/7 observation, assessment and treatment for children, that for teenagers, would often be undertaken as an inpatient.

- Work with the family and foster parental care.
- Wide range of assessment and treatment packages can be offered intensively.
- The partial 'therapeutic milieu' of the day unit shares care with family or local school to a greater extent than residential units. Thus, there are more opportunities for staff

to spend therapeutic time with parents and families; and likewise, a day unit can deliver treatment programmes that link closely with parent-based care.

- There are also opportunities to transfer learned skills into the community and family setting (McCarthy et al. 2006) or to provide outreach into the community.
- Day services cost less per young person treated than inpatient services, thereby potentially providing a more cost-effective alternative.

Disadvantages

- A day service may function as a 'cut down' version of inpatient care for districts that do not have an inpatient unit or block contract with an inpatient provider.
- Rigidity of programmes offered – whilst modernised day programmes offer the best of individually tailored bundles of care for young people, older-style day units may still offer rigidly set 'all inclusive' programmes, in which young people attend groups and activities that are not necessarily helpful for their particular difficulties, with little thought put into ensuring all interventions offered are evidence-based.
- Lack of opportunities to generalise learning and experience to young person's home and community.
- Many day units cannot provide a full educational programme, which may not enable the young person to achieve their academic goals, particularly where they are already failing in school. A day programme has to provide adequate academic input as well as a peer group and therapeutic experience. This is more easily achieved in an inpatient setting.
- The child may have to adapt to being in different environments (e.g. own school, pupil referral unit, home, respite care) during the week and in many areas the daily trip to and from the day programme may be long and tiring.
- The opportunities for completeness and intensity of treatment and observation are limited.
- Loss of income and transport costs may be substantial for some families who are not all entitled to benefits.

What does a day programme look like?

Young people attend a centre or unit one to five days a week for a day that may be as long as 8 a.m. to 8 p.m. (e.g. for an eating disorder day programme where all meals are supported) or as short as a school day (e.g. for assessment of neuro-developmental disorders). The day is structured with a timetable. There is usually a 'meet and greet' and 'debrief' session initially followed by a series of education sessions and therapeutic groups, interspersed by break times and meals. Meals and snacks are provided, with the young people and staff eating together. A brief plenary meeting to close the day may be held (see Box 4.4).

Individualised programmes may fit within the day however, and young people may leave part of the programme to attend their own school, or go for specialised assessments or individual and family therapy sessions. Thus a complex matrix of tailored individual packages fitting into a timetabled structure needs to be delivered by the staff team. Therapeutic milieu and therapeutic alliance need to be facilitated alongside practical considerations and both do appear to influence outcome (Hougaard 1994; Kroll & Green 1997; Grizenko 1997; Green 2006).

BOX 4.4 An example day programme

08.00–08.15	Arrival and Meet and Greet Group
08:15–09:00	Breakfast
09:00–10:00	Education on day programme or own school
10:00–11:00	Motivational group
11:00–11:30	Snack and break
11:30–13:00	Shopping group for evening meal or emotional regulation group and own time
13:00–14:00	Lunch
14:00–15:00	Education
15:00–15:45	Mindfulness group/Care Programme Approach (CPA) meeting/health clinic
15:45–16:15	Snack break
16:15–17:00	Cooking group or creative group
17:00–18:00	Homework club
18:00–18:45	Dinner
18:45–19.45	Family therapy/individual session
19.45–20.00	Family and young people closing session with keyworker

---

Staff have many different roles at different times, or even concurrently, with a young person and their family, including educator, therapist and collaborator with parent. Robust supervision is needed at individual clinician level, but also as a group, to ensure that the boundaries of care are clear and maintained. The risk otherwise is of a staff team replicating pre-existing parental splits, or delivering poor parenting with alternating punitive or lax boundaries.

Assessment processes

Working with young people on a daily basis for several hours a day gives great opportunities for detailed assessment of biological and psychological aspects of disorder. Assessment may be naturalistic or structured and there is room for both in the day programme setting.

Naturalistic

Close observation of a young person's features, and their manner of walking, talking and socially interacting may all suggest previously unrecognised underlying disorders. These may include congenital syndromes, undiagnosed complex seizures or unrecognised autistic spectrum conditions.

Structured

Day services, like inpatient units, need to be able to access a wide range of biological investigations. These include computed tomography (CT) and magnetic resonance imaging (MRI) scanning, as well as electroencephalography (EEG) and haematology and biochemistry investigations. In practice this means having staff trained in venepuncture, or access to local facilities. Developmental assessments such as structured speech and language assessments; occupational therapy (activities of daily living, assessment movement batteries); cognitive assessment such as psychometric evaluation; educational assessment (Performance Indicators for value Added Target Setting (PIVAT) scales, Standardised Assessment Tests (SATS) levels, contribution to assessment for statement of special educational needs (SEN)); and access to paediatric and neurological assessments may all be required by the day service team.

The linking of these different parts of the assessment is crucial to providing an integrated formulation. Some day services have structured assessment protocols in which different staff members of the clinical team have agreed tasks or roles (Green 2006). Staff will use specific skills from their core profession as well as generic skills (Green & Worrall-Davies 2008). This can be a complicated process and one which needs careful handling. Initial assumptions based on limited information, often gathered when the child or young person was in universal services, or community CAMHS, may be challenged in the context of new perspectives derived from the multidisciplinary day programme team.

Working in the day unit setting

Behavioural management is fundamental to ensure safe assessment and treatment. Policies and procedures must be in place to manage difficult or challenging behaviours such as aggression, bullying, self-harm or harm to others, and absconding. Staff must be trained to undertake verbal de-escalation techniques and in the use of physical restraint (American Academy of Child and Adolescent Psychiatry 2010). A thorough initial risk assessment and care planning undertaken collaboratively with the young person and their family minimises problems. Regular audit and self-assessment within a national group such as the Quality Network for Inpatient CAMHS (QNIC) may improve the quality of day unit care and protect against the isolation that day services may experience.

The staff team

As treatment approaches become more sophisticated the staff team in a day programme must deliver highly skilled interventions in the context of a time limited admission and increased throughput in and out of a valuable but expensive CAMHS resource. The American Academy of Child and Adolescent Psychiatry (2010) and the Royal College of Psychiatrists (1999) both emphasise the wide range of professional disciplines that should be represented in day units. Whilst most day programmes are delivered primarily by a nursing team, child and adolescent psychiatrists, social workers, clinical child psychologists, speech and language therapists, occupational therapists, physiotherapists, family therapists and child psychotherapists all have important roles.

Attempts to operate with too few staff are a recipe for stress, burnout and institutional decay. The American Academy of Child and Adolescent Psychiatry (AACAP) recommends that young people are seen weekly by their psychiatrist, and that their exit strategy is planned right from admission, and that meetings within a care planning framework happen at least monthly. Models of team functioning vary with the purpose and setting of the day service. A popular current style is staff working generically in a team, with a flat hierarchy, with task-focused 'mini teams' (Green & Worrall-Davies 2008).

Do day programmes work?

Research comparing day units historically has been problematic to undertake, because they offer such varied programmes and work to different treatment models. No randomised controlled study has been undertaken for day services alone. More recent evidence has focused on day programmes for specific disorders rather than controlled studies. Innovative examples of day services provide opportunities to transfer care and treatment from inpatient settings into the community and family environment (McCarthy et al. 2006), or meet the needs of children and young people with complex needs through multi-agency partnerships between health, education and social services.

Day programmes and conduct disorder

Children and young people with unsocialised aggressive or disruptive behaviours who are admitted to inpatient services consistently have poor outcomes (Green et al. 2007) reflecting the general poor prognosis for such disorders. However, a classic controlled study of day treatment versus waiting list showed that the day programme was effective for preschool and school age children with severe behaviour problems (Grizenko et al. 1993a, 1993b). Improvements in behaviour, self-esteem and self-reported mood were significantly greater than those seen in the waiting list group, both at discharge and at six-month follow-up. However, the sample size was small with only 15 children in each group.

The five-year follow-up of these same children (Grizenko 1997) found that compared to pre-treatment, a significantly greater number were in mainstream education. A small proportion (9 per cent) of children required further CAMHS input after discharge from the day programme, including re-admission to a day programme or admission to an inpatient unit. Nearly a fifth (18 per cent) required social care input including temporary residential placement. Poor parental cooperation during the day programme predicted likelihood of requiring social care or CAMHS input after discharge from the day programme. Normal range intelligence quotient (IQ) score and good parental involvement predicted a positive five-year outcome.

Another multi-modal day programme (Rey et al. 1998) also showed improvement over matched controls who had received other treatments; however, neither group had a good outcome overall.

Day programmes and eating disorders

In a systematic review of 39-day programmes for eating disorders in adults, Zipfel and colleagues (2002) found that although there were major global differences in healthcare settings and aims, the mainstay of treatment in most was group based. In the last decade, the treatment of young people with eating disorders has focused on the development of individual work with a motivational or cognitive behavioural therapy (CBT) based focus, and on multi-family-based therapy embedded in the day programme setting. Goldstein et al. (2010) reported significant weight gain and clinically important changes in attitude toward eating and food in a group of young people both at discharge and at six-month follow-up after completion of a ten-week day-based 'transition program' which included considerable family-based therapy as well as motivational and CBT-based strategies

In the multi-family day treatment model families work together on the problem of living with young people with an eating disorder (Eisler 2005). There is intensive attendance over several days. Families are encouraged to explore how the eating disorder and the patterns of communication in the family have become entangled, and how this has led to difficulties for the family in 'getting back on track'. The sharing of experiences between families and the intensity of the programme, together with the emphasis on helping families find their own solutions are the day programme's unique features (Dare & Eisler 2000; Scholz & Asen 2001).

There is little efficacy evidence yet, but preliminary results suggest that there is significant symptomatic improvement (Fairbairn & Eisler 2007) and that family satisfaction with the treatment model is high and drop-out rates are low (Scholz et al. 2005). Rockwell and colleagues (2011) report a small initial case series ($n = 19$) using this model. All but one young person had sustained post-treatment weight gain (mean = 15.0, SD = +/- 14.5). A multi-centre randomised controlled trial is currently being evaluated.

Day programmes and substance misuse

Cornwall & Blood (1998) compared the efficacy of inpatient versus day patient treatment for substance abuse in 135 Canadian adolescents. Young people in both arms of the study were multiple drug abusers. Both groups received a primary group intervention which included psycho-education, skills development, psychotherapy and schooling on site. The day treatment programme was offered five days per week for ten weeks. Treatment completion rates were found to be similar between both groups with similar reductions in substance use, behaviour difficulties, and better functioning as measured using a battery of standardised measures.

Day programmes and psychosis

There are no efficacy studies but Clark (2001) suggests that young people with psychosis may be managed as day patients, with key determinants being level of risk to self or others, degree of psychosocial complexity, and the likely compliance and engagement with investigation and treatment.

The modern day service in the wider multi-agency setting

Integrated inpatient and day units can share programming, staff and infrastructure. The advantages of independent day units relate to flexibility. The reduced need for a shift system to cover nights allows nursing staff to work predictable hours and be available regularly to contribute to liaison sessions and outreach work. Partial attendance also means that the staff group has time for supervision and continuing professional development and educational activities. The flexibility of inpatient, day and outreach services is emerging as a priority. Street (2004) highlighted the need for more CAMHS to be able to offer outreach and/or day care before and after admission.

As care pathways become the mainstay of CAMHS, and in line with NICE guidance, mental healthcare for young people now is less loosely multi-modal and much more streamlined. Treatments are focused more on tailored individual care, incorporating patient and family choice, and following evidence-based care pathways for each condition or problem area. This means that the old style 'one size fits all' day units have realigned themselves to fit with new ways of working in CAMHS. More day programmes are now offering assessment and evidence-based interventions for specific conditions such as autism spectrum conditions. Others are closely aligning with alternative 'wraparound' services to provide seamless care between community services, outreach and inpatient care. This is as part of planned care pathways designed to prevent crisis admissions.

Treatment goals and outcomes

Shaw (1998) described the use of treatment goal planning, which is especially useful with young people with complex needs such as those in day services. Staff thinking, and treatment planning are kept focused and therapeutic 'drift' is reduced. Treatment goals should be specific, measurable, achievable, realistic and timely (SMART) and ideally framed in the child's own words. Such aims or goals should also be flexible so that they can change if needed during treatment.

Rothery et al. (1995) audited treatment goals in young people admitted to four adolescent units. They found that the majority of treatment goals included a wide range of aims. These included those focused on improving relationships and achieving developmental or maturational targets rather than just changes in symptoms. Improvements in all these goals occurred during treatment. Over a decade later, the CAMHS Outcome Research Consortium (CORC) includes 'goal-based outcomes (GBO)' in its suggested suite of outcome measures. These are highly suitable for day programme use since they measure outcomes across a broad spectrum of interventions, across a variety of settings, and with a variety of service users (Law 2009).

Preventing admissions

Intensive outreach and day programmes do not fully replace the need for inpatient beds but do prevent some admissions and reduce the duration of care in hospital. For example, the Leeds CAMHS outreach and Eating Disorder Day Programme (EDDP) are staffed by the same staff team. Bed stay in the local adolescent unit was reduced from 72 median days to 29 days over an 18-month period after the commissioning arrangements changed (Worrall-Davies et al. 2011a). With inpatient services costing several hundred pounds per day, admission alternatives such as day care and outreach services may provide a more cost-effective option that is attractive to commissioners and providers alike, as well as young people and their families.

A decade ago, O'Herlihy and colleagues (2003) found that a third of inpatient units are only open 5 days a week, and therefore could potentially be operating as day services. However, many now operate over 7 days, and both commissioners and providers must bear in mind that day services come at an additional cost to families (Green et al. 2007). This is because parents and carers may be required to transport their children to and from units at some distance from their homes, and at times that may require them to take significant time off work. Anecdotally, the Leeds Eating Disorder Day Programme (EDDP) has found that parents have found the financial and time burdens considerable, and in practice, transporting young people to the programme has been shared between family members and EDDP staff (Worrall-Davies et al. 2011b).

Raising the age threshold to 18 or even 25 years in response to the increase in severe mental illness presenting in young teenagers, the recommendations from the Office of the Children's Commissioner (2007) and the 'Age Appropriate Environment' amendment (section 131a of the Mental Health Act) 2007 may be helpful for the complex groups of young people who attend day and other intensive community CAMHS provision.

Summary and conclusions

Nowadays, with a wide range of alternatives to inpatient care in CAMHS and new commissioning demands, day programmes have had to focus clearly on what they deliver and to whom and with what effect. Most day services now deliver one or more discrete functions, usually in relation to a 'step-up, step-down' approach, or offer assessment and targeted treatment packages for children and young people with specific disorders. Such care packages typically comprise targeted, five day-a-week interventions offering multi-modal 'bundles', of individual, family and psychopharmacological interventions alongside intensive family therapy and parenting work.

The main advantages and disadvantages of day services need to be considered. Costs to the family can be great in terms of disruption to work and financial costs of travel and parking, compared to intensive community services, where the corresponding travel costs are borne by the NHS.

The evidence for the clinical effectiveness of day services is mixed and much dates back to when day services were generic. It is therefore difficult to extrapolate findings to the current system, or indeed to extrapolate to day service in other countries, as day programmes in North America, the UK and Australasia are vastly different. However, for conduct disorder, follow up at six months and five years suggests continuing reduction of symptoms.

Research in the last decade suggests that day programmes incorporating motivational and CBT-based strategies, or those based on the multiple family day treatment model have positive outcomes. Although there is little formal research, young people with substance misuse and psychosis are probably both helped by day services, and, certainly for psychosis, day care is as effective but clearly less restrictive and less disruptive than inpatient stay.

Modern day services need to be able to adapt to the changing NHS and changing CAMHS in a climate of financial restraint and austerity. Flexibility of approach and delivery, provision of individually tailored packages of evidence-based treatment and clear care planning are crucial. Evidence of adherence to local and national guidance, and quality standards also are crucial in the ever widening marketplace.

References

American Academy of Child and Adolescent Psychiatry. (2010). *Principles of Care for Treatment of Children and Adolescents with Mental Illnesses in Residential Treatment Centers.* http://www.aacap.org/galleries/defaultfile/Principles_of_Care_in_RTC_FINAL.pdf

Clark, A. (2001). Proposed treatment for adolescent psychosis. 1: Schizophrenia and schizophrenia-like psychoses. *Advances in Psychiatric Treatment*, 7, 16–23.

Cornwall, A. & Blood, L. (1998). Inpatient versus day treatment for substance abusing adolescents. *Journal of Nervous and Mental Disease*, 186, 580–582.

Dare, C. & Eisler, I. (2000). A multi-family group day treatment programme for adolescent eating disorder. *European Eating Disorders Review*, 8, 4–18.

Eisler, I. (2005). The empirical and theoretical base of family therapy and multiple family day therapy for adolescent anorexia nervosa. *Journal of Family Therapy*, 27, 104–131.

Ellilä, H., Sourander, A., Valimaki, M. & Piha, J. (2005). Characteristics and staff resources of child and adolescent psychiatric hospitals in Finland. *Journal of Psychiatric and Mental Health Nursing*, 12, 209–214.

Fairbairn, P. and Eisler, I. (2007). Thérapie multifamiliale intensive en unité de jour: groupe thérapeutique et groupe de formation. In S. Cook-Darzens (ed.) *Thérapies Multifamiliales Des Groupes Comme Agents Thérapeutiques /Multiple family therapy: groups as therapeutic agents.* (pp. 179–203). Paris: Éditions Érès.

Goldstein, M., Peters, L., Baillie, A., McVeagh, P., Minshell, G. & Fitzjames, D. (2011). The effectiveness of a day program for the treatment of adolescent anorexia nervosa, *International Journal of Eating Disorders,* 44, 29–38.

Green, J. (2006). The therapeutic alliance: a significant but neglected variable in child mental health treatment studies. *Journal of Child Psychology and Psychiatry*, 47, 425–435.

Green, J. & Jacobs, B. (1998). Current practice: a questionnaire survey of inpatient child psychiatry in the UK. In Green, J. M. & Jacobs, B. W. (Eds) *Inpatient Child Psychiatry: modern practice research and the future.* London: Routledge.

Green, J. & Worrall-Davies, A. (2008). Provision of intensive treatment, inpatient units, day units and intensive outreach. In Rutter, M., Hersov, L. & Taylor, E. (Eds) *Child and Adolescent Psychiatry: Modern Approaches*, 5th edition. Oxford: Blackwell.

Green, J., Jacobs, B., Beecham, J., Dunn, G., Kroll, L., Tobias, C. & Briskman, J. (2007). Inpatient treatment in child and adolescent psychiatry – a prospective study of health gain and costs. *Journal of Child Psychology and Psychiatry*, 48, 1259–1267.

Grizenko, N. (1997). Outcome of multimodal day treatment for children with severe behavior problems: a five-year follow up. *Journal of the American Academy of Child and Adolescent Psychiatry*, 36, 989–997.

Grizenko, N., Papineau, D. & Sayegh, L. (1993a). A comparison of day treatment and outpatient treatment for children with disruptive behavior problems. *Canadian Journal of Psychiatry*, 38, 432–435.

Grizenko, N., Papineau, D. & Sayegh, L. (1993b). Effectiveness of a multimodal day treatment program for children with disruptive behavior problems. *Journal of American Academy of Child and Adolescent Psychiatry*, 32, 127–134.

Hougaard, E. (1994). The therapeutic alliance: a conceptual analysis. *Scandinavian Journal of Psychology*, 35, 67–85.

Kroll, L. & Green, J. (1997). Therapeutic alliance in inpatient child psychiatry: development and initial validation of the Family Engagement Questionnaire. *Clinical Child Psychology and Psychiatry*, 2, 431–447.

Law, D. (2009). *Mind the Gap. Evidence-based interventions for children and families with more complex mental health needs.* http://www.newsavoypartnership.org/2009presentations/28_Duncan_Law_day_two_workshop_two.pdf

McCarthy, G., Baker, S., Betts, K., Bernard, D., Dove, J., Elliot, M., et al. (2006). The development of a new day treatment program for older children (8–11 years) with behavioural problems: The Go-Zone. *Clinical Child Psychology and Psychiatry*, 11, 156–166.

McDougall, T., Worrall-Davies, A., Hewson, L., Richardson, G. & Cotgrove, A. (2008). Tier 4 CAMHS – inpatient care, day services and alternatives: an overview of Tier 4 CAMHS provision in the UK. *Child and Adolescent Mental Health*, 13(4), 173–180.

O'Herlihy, A., Worrall, A., Lelliott, P., Jaffa, T., Hill, P. & Banerjee, S. (2003). Distribution and characteristics of in-patient child and adolescent mental health services in England and Wales. *British Journal of Psychiatry*, 183, 547–551.

Rey, J., Denshire, E., Wever, C. & Apollonov, I. (1998). Three year outcome of disruptive adolescents treated in a day program. *European Child and Adolescent Psychiatry*, 7, 42–48.

Rockwell, R., Boutelle, K., Trunko, M., Jacobs, M. & Kaye, W. (2011). An innovative short-term, intensive, family-based treatment for adolescent anorexia nervosa: case series. *European Eating Disorders Review*, 19(4) 362–367.

Rothery, D., Wrate, R., McCabe, R. & Aspin, J. (1995). Treatment goal planning: outcome findings of a British prospective multicentre study of adolescent inpatient units. *European Child and Adolescent Psychiatry*, 4, 209–220.

Royal College of Psychiatrists. (1999). *Guidance for the staffing of child and adolescent inpatient units.* Council Report 62. London: Royal College of Psychiatrists.

Scholz M. & Asen K. (2001). Multiple family therapy with eating disordered adolescents. *European Eating Disorders Review*, 9, 33–42.

Scholz, M., Rix, M., Scholz, K., Gantchev, K. and Thomke, V. (2005). Multiple family therapy for anorexia nervosa: concepts, experiences and results. *Journal of Family Therapy*, 27(2), 132–141.

Shaw, M. (1998). Childhood mental health and the law. In Green, J. M. & Jacobs, B. W. (Eds) *Inpatient Child Psychiatry: modern practice, research and the future* (pp. 349–362). London: Routledge.

Street, C. (2004). Inpatient mental health services for young people: changing to meet new needs? *Journal of the Royal Society for the Promotion of Health*, 124, 115–118.

Worrall-Davies, A., Ross, E & Robinson, J. (2011). Personal communication 1 October 2011. Transport of young people to and from the Leeds EDDP.

Worrall-Davies, A., Beal, H., Ferguson, L. and Ross E. (2011). *Interim evaluation of CAMH Outreach and Therapies Service.* Leeds Community Healthcare NHS Trust: unpublished audit.

Zipfel, S., Reas, D., Thornton, C., Olmsted, M., Williamson, D., Gerlinghoff, M., Herzog, W. & Beumont, P. (2002). Day hospitalization programs for eating disorders: a systematic review of the literature. *International Journal of Eating Disorders*, 31, 105–117.

5

EARLY INTERVENTION PSYCHOSIS SERVICES FOR YOUNG PEOPLE WITH PSYCHOSIS

Tim McDougall

Key points

- Intensive community, hospital and home-based services for children and young people should be configured to facilitate early detection and treatment of psychosis and schizophrenia.
- There is very little evidence about which service model works best for children and young people with psychosis and schizophrenia. There are no randomised controlled trials or systematic reviews investigating CAMHS or early intervention in psychosis (EIP) services and many other studies are limited in their scope and design and age group being considered.
- The primary role of general practitioners (GPs) and primary care professionals in the care and treatment of children and young people with psychosis or schizophrenia is in relation to physical health monitoring. This is due to the heightened risk of obesity and complications of this such as diabetes and cardiovascular disease and other health problems associated with psychotic disorders.
- EIP services provide community level interventions for people aged between 14 and 35 who are in the early phase of psychosis or schizophrenia. EIP teams offer specialised psychosocial and pharmacological interventions, and increasingly use a 'recovery' model to help optimise social, education and vocational outcomes.
- The NICE guidance on psychosis and schizophrenia in children and young people suggests that a specialist early intervention approach may offer advantages over generic community CAMHS.
- Children and young people with psychosis or schizophrenia should usually only be admitted to hospital if the risks associated with their care and treatment make management at community level unsafe, or they require intensive 24-hour nursing care. This is because hospital admission can have a negative impact on family life, education and social relationships.

Introduction

Schizophrenia has been identified as the ninth leading cause of disability among all known diseases and it is the most persistent and disabling of all the major mental disorders (Murray & Lopez 1996). This chapter explores what we mean by psychosis and schizophrenia; discusses approaches to assessment and treatment; and describes how services are organised and provided for children, young people and their families.

Children and young people with psychosis or schizophrenia do not necessarily require hospital admission. On the contrary, the majority of children and young people can be appropriately and successfully supported by community CAMHS or EIP services. The role and function of these services are described in this chapter along with a discussion about when treatment in hospital may be required.

What do we mean by psychosis and schizophrenia?

Schizophrenia and psychosis in children and young people refers to a major psychiatric disorder or cluster of disorders characterised by positive psychotic symptoms such as hallucinations, delusions and thought disorder; and negative symptoms such as loss of motivation and social withdrawal.

No common cause of psychosis and schizophrenia has been identified in all children and young people. However, there is general consensus that these conditions result from a combination of genetic factors and life events. The stress–vulnerability model (Zubin & Spring 1977) is a way of understanding how the symptoms of psychosis and schizophrenia are developed and maintained. Some propose that due to the timing of onset, psychosis and schizophrenia can be understood as a disorder of adolescence and the consequence of severe disruption in this normally difficult psychological maturational process in vulnerable individuals (Harrop & Trower 2001).

A number of terms should be defined for the purposes of this chapter and in describing services for children and young people with psychosis or schizophrenia. These include what has historically been referred to as the 'prodromal' or 'at risk' mental state; 'early intervention'; the concept of 'duration of untreated psychosis'; and the principle of 'recovery'.

Early intervention

Whilst the significance of intervening early in the course of psychosis and schizophrenia has been acknowledged for over 70 years (Cameron 1938; McGorry 1998), a growing body of research evidence has continued to demonstrate the efficacy of early detection and intervention in helping to produce positive outcomes and recovery for people living with this condition (McGorry 1998; McGorry et al. 2002).

The phrase 'early intervention' is used in two ways when discussing children and young people with psychosis or schizophrenia. First, it refers to the principle of intervention at the earliest stage in order to optimise outcomes. Since children and young people with this condition have greater cognitive, psychological and social impairments, early detection and intervention is crucially important. Second, it is used to described 'early intervention services' which are discussed later in this chapter.

At risk mental states

The early stages of psychosis are sometimes referred to as the 'prodromal' phase which is a stage that may precede the onset of psychosis or schizophrenia. However, the term 'prodrome' is non-specific and ambiguous, and can only be applied after the psychotic stage develops. Consequently, the NICE guideline on schizophrenia and psychosis in children and young people (National Institute for Health and Clinical Excellence 2013) refers to 'at risk mental states', in an attempt to improve early detection and intervention. This of course assumes that it is possible to detect people at risk of psychosis, that their 'at risk' presentation will transition to psychosis, and that interventions will interrupt this trajectory.

Sometimes children and young people experience transient or 'attenuated' psychotic symptoms. Most do not go on to develop psychosis or schizophrenia but all should be assessed by a specialist mental health service and the urgency of this should be informed by any associated distress or impairment. Further research is required to establish whether attenuated psychotic symptoms and 'at risk' states predict young people who will and will not go on to develop psychosis and schizophrenia.

Duration of untreated psychosis

The Early Psychosis Declaration, supported by the World Health Organization (WHO), highlighted the need to reduce long delays in access to treatment that many people with psychosis and schizophrenia experience by better joint working and early intervention (Rethink/National Institute for Mental Health in England 2004).

The duration of untreated psychosis (DUP) refers to the period between the onset of symptoms and the start of appropriate treatment for those symptoms (Marshall et al. 2005). A longer DUP is strongly associated with poor outcomes (Johnstone et al. 1986; Birchwood et al. 1998) which was the evidence base on which the UK EIP services were developed. EIP services have been shown to reduce the DUP associated with schizophrenia and psychosis, as well as reduce hospital admissions and relapse rates (Bird et al. 2010). Policy guidance for EIP services specifies that the DUP is reduced to a service median of less than three months and an individual maximum of less than six months (Department of Health 2003).

Recovery

Early recovery appears to be an important indicator of outcome. Hollis & Rapoport (2011) report that adolescents who remain psychotic after 6 months of onset have only a 15 per cent chance of achieving full remission, whilst half of those who make a full recovery have psychotic symptoms for less than three months.

Service provision for young people with psychosis and schizophrenia

There is very little evidence about which service model works best for children and young people with psychosis and schizophrenia. There are no randomised controlled trials or systematic reviews investigating CAMHS or EIP services and many other studies are limited in their scope and design and age group being considered.

There is a lack of research comparing admission with alternative service provision for young people with psychosis and schizophrenia. However, studies of early intervention, many of which include young people under the age of 18, report that intensive care in the community can be at least as effective as admission (Spencer et al. 2001).

Primary care services

GPs are often the first point of contact for children and young people with suspected psychosis or schizophrenia. In a study of primary care, a third of 13- to 16-year-olds attending their GP had evidence of a current or previous psychiatric disorder including psychosis or schizophrenia (Kramer & Garralda 2000). The NICE guidance advises GPs to refer a child or young person who has sustained psychotic symptoms lasting four weeks or more to specialist CAMHS or EIP services (National Institute for Health and Clinical Excellence 2013).

The primary role of GPs and primary care professionals in the care and treatment of psychosis or schizophrenia is in relation to physical health monitoring for children and young people on medication. This is due to the heightened risk of obesity and complications of this such as diabetes and cardiovascular disease and other health problems associated with psychotic disorders. The NICE guidance recommends that secondary care professionals should monitor and manage any side effects associated with antipsychotic medication (National Institute for Health and Clinical Excellence 2013). If it is necessary for a GP to start antipsychotic medication they should have experience in treating and managing schizophrenia. Children and young people who are receiving ongoing treatment in primary care may need to be referred to specialist services if they become unwell or the risks to themselves or others increase.

Community CAMHS

It has been suggested that due to the relative rarity of psychosis and schizophrenia in children and young people, Tier 3 CAMHS teams may not be able to provide the full range of evidence-based treatments required, particularly for those aged over 16. These may include outreach, home-based intervention and psychosocial interventions. The NICE guidance on psychosis and schizophrenia in children and young people suggests that a specialist early intervention approach may offer advantages over generic community CAMHS due to the concentration of skills, experience and resources in EIP teams.

EIP services

EIP services originated in the NHS Plan published in 2000. They were intended to provide community level interventions for people aged between 14 and 35 who are in prodromal and early phase of psychosis or schizophrenia (Department of Health 2001). The model of care that has evolved is based on the principles of 'assertive outreach' and is now part of healthcare provision across the UK, Europe and North America. Engagement with families is an important element, particularly for children and young people who are may be living with parents or carers. EIP teams offer specialised psychosocial and pharmacological interventions, and increasingly use a 'recovery' model to help optimise social, education and vocational outcomes.

To help implement the National Service Framework (NSF) for Mental Health (Department of Health 1999) the Government published guidance on implementing EIP services (Department of Health 2001). This stated that CAMHS and adult mental health services should work together with commissioners to ensure that all young people aged 14 to 35 years with a first episode of psychosis receive early intervention by a designated early psychosis service. Key requirements of these EIP services were to:

- reduce the length of time that young people remain undiagnosed and untreated;
- provide a seamless service available for those from age 14 to 35 that effectively integrates child, adolescent and adult mental health services and works in partnership with primary care, education, social services, youth and other services;
- develop meaningful engagement, provide evidence-based interventions and promote recovery during the early phase of illness;
- increase stability in the lives of service users, facilitate development and provide opportunities for personal fulfilment;
- ensure that the care is transferred thoughtfully and effectively at the end of the treatment period; and
- reduce stigma associated with psychosis and improve professional and lay awareness of the symptoms of psychosis and the need for early intervention.

Children and young people with psychosis or schizophrenia who are being treated in an EIP service should have access to that service for up to three years (or until their 18th birthday, whichever period is longer) regardless of the age of onset of psychosis or schizophrenia (National Institute for Health and Clinical Excellence 2013).

Despite policy and associated guidance, the roles and responsibilities of CAMHS and EIP teams for local children and young people with psychosis and schizophrenia vary across the country (Rethink 2011). The majority of UK EIP teams form part of adult mental health services and only a minority are located in CAMHS. In 2004 a group of international experts published a report on the essential elements of EIP services and their relationship with CAMHS. There was consensus that the two services should be integrated, and that EIP should employ youth workers and have dedicated input from a child and adolescent psychiatrist (Marshall et al. 2004). In practice, however, audits have shown that only a minority of EIP teams include input from CAMHS and, despite the national guidance (Department of Health 2001), some do not see young people under 16 at all (Pinfold et al. 2007).

Effectiveness of EIP services

There is evidence that EIP services are not only clinically and cost effective (National Institute for Health and Clinical Excellence 2013), but current national mental health policy cites them as a vital part of shifting the focus of services towards prevention and early identification and intervention (Department of Health 2011). The national mental health strategy, *No Health without Mental Health* (Department of Health 2011), states that EIP services for young people aged 14–35 with the first onset of psychosis have been shown to benefit individuals, reduce relapse, improve employment and educational outcomes, and reduce risk of suicide and homicide.

In their briefing on early intervention services, the NHS Confederation (2011) suggests that EIP services offer mental health providers opportunities to support the delivery of key objectives within the mental health strategy. The Confederation adds that through their innovative practice, EIP services have evidenced substantial clinical improvements; met productivity targets; reduced costs; and, most importantly, have been well received by the clients, families and the referral agencies that have experienced them.

Hospital care

Until the early 1990s most adolescents with psychosis and schizophrenia were admitted to inpatient CAMHS units. This was partly because there were very few alternatives and EIP teams were not in existence. Community CAMHS often stopped working with children at 16 which is the point when the incidence of psychotic disorders increases (Kirkbride et al. 2006).

Children and young people with psychosis or schizophrenia should usually only be admitted to hospital if the risks associated with their care and treatment make management at community level unsafe, or they require intensive 24-hour nursing care. This is because hospital admission can have a negative impact on family life, education and social relationships (Milin et al. 2000). It can compromise the mastery of developmental tasks of adolescence such as separating from parents, increasing autonomy and forming a supportive peer network. The NICE (2013) guidance on psychosis and schizophrenia points out that hospital admission can be disruptive and inpatient admission should be seen as one part of a care pathway rather than an end in itself. There should be close liaison and collaboration with community CAMHS and EIP services, and the Care Programme Approach (CPA) should be the framework that supports this.

Admission to hospital in crisis should be to an appropriate hospital environment which is usually an adolescent unit. There may be occasions when an adult ward is more appropriate than a CAMHS unit. This might be where the young person is experiencing a first episode of psychosis and their care in hospital is likely to go beyond their 18th birthday. However, a young person's care on an adult ward should take account of their developmental needs. In some areas of the UK access to adolescent hospital beds is limited. For example, a Scottish survey of first episode presentations by adolescents found that 80 per cent were hospitalised on adult wards, suggesting that most had reached crisis before accessing services (Boeing et al. 2007).

Discharge from hospital must be carefully planned in conjunction with community services. The transition from hospital to CAMHS or EIP services should be supported as this is a time of vulnerability for relapse.

Assessment

Whether a child or young person is being assessed in CAMHS or EIP services some general principles apply. The assessment should be multidisciplinary and comprehensive and undertaken by those with skills and competencies in psychosis and schizophrenia and working with children and young people. The assessment should be paced according to the child or young person's level of understanding, emotional maturity and cognitive abilities. The following areas of need should be addressed during the assessment:

• developmental history;
• mental health and disorder including co-morbidity;
• psychological and psychosocial functioning;
• functioning in education, training or employment;
• physical health and history;
• family needs.

Parents and carers

The parents or carers of children and young people with psychosis or schizophrenia usually have a key role to play and should be involved according to the age and wishes of their child or young person. If the child is Gillick competent they should be asked what can and cannot be shared with their parents or carers.

Treatment

Treatments for children and young people with psychosis or schizophrenia are psychological, pharmacological, psychosocial, psycho-educational or, most commonly, a combination of all these modalities. Within the scope of this chapter it is not possible to describe the full range of interventions that are available as well as a discussion of the evidence or lack of evidence for such treatments. Therefore some general principles as well as information in relation to where the evidence is most strong (or less weak) are discussed.

Antipsychotic medication

Depending which antipsychotic medication to use depends on a range of factors including patient choice, the relative risks of extra pyramidal side effects (EPSE), metabolic side effects and other adverse events which the child or young person may find unpleasant or difficult to tolerate. The decision about which drug to use should be made in partnership between the child or young person, their parents or carers and clinicians.

Baseline assessments and monitoring

Before starting a child or young person on antipsychotic medication it is best practice to perform baseline investigations. Weight and height should be plotted on a growth chart, and waist and hip circumference should be recorded on a percentile chart. An electrocardiogram (ECG) is recommended, particularly if there is a family history of cardiovascular disease.

Table 5.1 summarises the assessments that NICE recommend before starting children and young people on antipsychotic medication. This should be considered in conjunction with guidance from the British National Formulary (BNF), British National Formulary for Children (BNFC) and the summary of product characteristics (SPC) for the medications concerned.

Initial treatment of psychosis or schizophrenia with antipsychotic medication should be considered as an individual therapeutic trial. The indications for treatment and the anticipated benefits and risks should be discussed with the child or young person as well as their parents and carers. The dose should be at the lower end of the licensed range and

TABLE 5.1   Baseline investigations and monitoring for children and young people who are prescribed antipsychotic medication

	Investigations at baseline	Weekly monitoring in first 6 weeks	Monitor at 12 weeks	Monitor every 6 months thereafter	Monitor throughout treatment and particularly during titration
Weight	✓	✓	✓	✓	
Height	✓			✓	
Waist and hip circumference	✓			✓	
Pulse	✓		✓	✓	
Blood pressure	✓		✓	✓	
Fasting blood glucose	✓		✓	✓	
Glycosylated haemoglobin	✓		✓	✓	
Blood lipids	✓		✓	✓	
Prolactin	✓		✓	✓	
Movement disorders	✓				✓
Nutritional status	✓				✓
Tolerance of side effects	✓				
ECG	✓				
Efficacy					✓
Side effects					✓
Adherence					✓

Source: Adapted from National Institute for Health and Clinical Excellence (2013).

should be titrated slowly upwards. The efficacy should be monitored focusing specifically on symptoms and behaviour and side effects. Trials should be of 4- to 6-weeks duration and treatment should be at optimum dosage.

If a child or young person becomes acutely unwell and requires hospitalisation it may be necessary to use rapid tranquillisation, particularly if they present an imminent risk to themselves or others. In such circumstances clinicians should observe NICE guidance for the management of aggression and violence (National Institute for Health and Clinical Excellence 2005)

Psychological interventions

Psychological interventions are often set in the context of the stress–vulnerability model although this is not the only model to explain and treat people with psychosis and schizophrenia. Psycho-educational interventions based on the stress–vulnerability model have previously been described for use with children and families in primary care settings (Asarnow et al. 2001). This intervention is designed to enhance understanding of symptoms through a working model that links stress to effects on feelings, thoughts and behaviour which if left unchallenged can lead to deterioration in mental health.

Research findings indicate that psychotic symptoms can be conceptualised with reference to normal psychological processes, and this then makes the content of symptoms understandable and suitable for cognitive behavioural therapy (CBT) interventions (e.g. Chadwick et al., 1996). However, there is little evidence that psychological interventions for psychotic symptoms are effective without medication. The NICE guidance suggests that CBT may be helpful as an adjunct to antipsychotic medication for both symptom reduction and relapse prevention. This is by supporting the child or young person to link their thoughts, feelings and behaviours and appraise and monitor these in the context of their current or past experiences. This may enable them to re-evaluate perceptions or challenge unhelpful beliefs and reduce anxiety or distress. However, it is important to note that the evidence base for CBT derives largely from randomised controlled trials conducted in adult populations.

Like all treatments, psychological interventions should be planned and delivered collaboratively. Any psychological intervention, including CBT, should be developmentally appropriate to the age and understanding of the child or young person. In practice, this involves adapting adult models to suit the needs of children and young people. However, not all children and young people can work with a CBT model.

Children and young people with psychosis or schizophrenia have often had experiences of trauma (Read et al. 2005; Kilcommons & Morrison 2005; Morrison 2009). It is important that the treatment programme includes psychotherapeutic interventions where these are indicated. Providing this separately can be problematic and may lead to fragmented care.

The importance of good care planning

Children and young people with psychosis use primary, secondary and tertiary level health services and receive care and treatment in hospital and community settings. In order to help ensure continuity of access, and to avoid unhelpful transitions, care and treatment should be carefully planned and organised. For example, children and young people who are taking antipsychotic medication are at heightened risk of adverse events (Kumra et al. 2008) and responsibility for physical care, baseline assessments and monitoring needs to be clear to all those involved in the care plan.

The NICE guidance on service user experience of adult mental health has been adapted to the needs of children and young people. This states that children and young people with psychosis or schizophrenia should be routinely able to access care from a single multidisciplinary team, are not passed from one team to another and do not undergo multiple assessments (National Institute for Health and Clinical Excellence 2013).

Crisis plans

The care plan for a child or young person with psychosis or schizophrenia should always include a crisis element. This should be developed in conjunction with the young person, their parents or carers and professionals involved in the care package. This is so that intervention in crisis is timely and hospital admission is avoided wherever possible. The crisis plan should include 'relapse signatures' or signs that a young person may be becoming unwell, details of the support network to help prevent hospital admission and the roles, responsibilities and contact details of all professional who are involved.

Depending on the age of the child or young person and where they live, services may be available to help avoid hospital admission. For young people over 16, crisis resolution and home treatment (CRHT) teams are usually available where support can be provided in the community or at home. For children under 16 the options are much more limited. There are very few crisis resolution and home treatment teams in CAMHS, and children in psychiatric crisis are usually admitted to hospital where facilities for emergency admission exist. However, not all adolescent units have the capacity, capability or willingness to admit young people in an emergency, which means they sometimes get admitted to inappropriate settings such as paediatric wards, adult mental health wards or police custody (McDougall & Bodley-Scott 2008).

Staff training and development

Professionals should be trained, skilled and competent to work with children and young people who have psychosis or schizophrenia. They should be aware of legislation such as the Children Act 1989, Mental Health Act 1983 and the Mental Capacity Act 2005. Due to the risks of self-neglect and harm young people may pose to themselves or others, staff must be familiar with safeguarding policies and procedures. Whilst a range of professions and skills help produce good outcomes in EIP services, Brooker & Repper (2001) suggest that the relationships, attitudes and interpersonal skills are also vital for the success of the team. Where healthcare professionals are providing psychological treatments for children, young people and families they should have achieved an appropriate level of competence to deliver the intervention and have access to a competent and experienced clinical supervisor.

Summary

The NICE (2013) guidance on psychosis and schizophrenia suggests that a good experience of care for children and young people is underpinned by effective interventions delivered safely by competent professionals in the appropriate service. This chapter has discussed some of the psychological and pharmacological treatments that are available and the services that deliver them.

References

Asarnow, J., Jaycox, L. & Thompson, M. (2001). Depression in youth: psychosocial interventions. *Journal of Clinical Child Psychology*, 30(1), 33–47.

Birchwood, M., Todd, P. & Jackson, C. (1998). Early intervention in psychosis: the critical period hypothesis. *British Journal of Psychiatry*, 172, 53–59.

Bird, V., Premkumar, P. & Kendall, T. (2010). Early intervention services, cognitive behavioural therapy and family therapy in early psychosis: systemic review. *British Journal of Psychiatry*, 197, 350–356.

Boeing, L., Murray, V. & Pelosi, A. (2007). Adolescent onset psychosis: prevalence, needs and service provision. *British Journal of Psychiatry*, 190, 18–26.

Brooker, C. & Repper, J. (2001). *Serious Mental Health Problems in the Community: policy, practice and research*. London: Baillière Tindall.

Cameron, D. (1938). Early schizophrenia. *American Journal of Psychiatry*, (95), 567–578.

Chadwick, P., Birchwood, M. & Trower, P. (1996). *Cognitive Therapy of Delusions, Voices and paranoia*. Chichester: John Wiley and Sons.

Department of Health. (2011). *No Health without Mental Health: a cross government mental health outcomes strategy for people of all ages*. London: HMSO.

Department of Health. (2003). *Early Intervention for People with Psychosis: expert briefing*. London: HMSO.

Department of Health. (2001). *Policy Implementation Guidance for Early Intervention Services*. London: HMSO.

Department of Health. (1999). *National Service Framework for Mental Health*. London: HMSO.

Harrop, C. & Trower, P. (2001). Why does schizophrenia develop at late adolescence? *Clinical Psychology Review*, 21(2), 241–265.

Hollis, C. & Rapaport, J. (2011). Child and adolescent schizophrenia. In: Weinberger, D. & Harrison, P. (eds). *Schizophrenia* (3rd edition), Wiley: London.

Johnstone, E., Crow, T. & Johnson. A. (1986). The Northwick Park studies of first episodes of schizophrenia. 1: presentation of the illness and problems relating to admission. *British Journal of Psychiatry*, 148, 115–120.

Kilcommons, A. & Morrison, A.P. (2005). Relationships between trauma and psychosis: an exploration of cognitive and dissociative factors. *Acta Psychiatrica Scandinavica*, 112(5), 351–359.

Kirkbride, J., Fearon, P. & Morgan, C. (2006). Heterogeneity in incidence rates of schizophrenia and other psychotic syndromes: findings from the 3-center AeSOP study. *Archives of General Psychiatry*, 63, 250–258.

Kramer, T. & Garralda, M. (2000). Child and adolescent mental health problems in primary care. *Advances in Psychiatric Treatment*, 6, 287–294.

Kumra, S., Oberstar, J. & Sikich, L. (2008). Efficacy and tolerability of second generation antipsychotics in children and adolescents with schizophrenia. *Schizophrenia Bulletin*, 34, 60–71.

McDougall, T. & Bodley-Scott, S. (2008). Too much too young: under 18s on adult mental health wards. *Mental Health Practice*, 11(6), 12–15.

McGorry, P. (1998). Preventative strategies in early psychosis: verging on reality. *British Journal of Psychiatry*, 172(33), 1–2.

McGorry, P.D., Yung, A.R., Phillips, L.J., Yuen, H.P., Francey, S., Cosgrave, E.M., et al. (2002). Randomized controlled trial of interventions designed to reduce the risk of progression to first-episode psychosis in a clinical sample with sub-threshold symptoms. *Archives of General Psychiatry*, 59, 921–928.

Marshall, M., Lewis, S., Lockwood, A. & Drake, R. (2005). Association between duration of untreated psychosis and outcome in cohorts of first episode patients: a systematic review. *Archives of General Psychiatry*, 62(9), 975–983.

Marshall, M., Lockwood, A. & Lewis, S. (2004). Essential elements of an early intervention service for psychosis: the opinions of expert clinicians. *BMC Psychiatry*, 4, 17.

Milin, R., Coupland, K.,Walker, S. & Fisher-Bloom, E. (2000). Outcome and follow-up study of an adolescent psychiatric day treatment school program. *Journal of the American Academy of Child and Adolescent Psychiatry*, 39, 320–328.

Morrison, A.P. (2009). A cognitive behavioural perspective on the relationship between childhood trauma and psychosis. *Epidemiologia e Psichiatria Sociale*, 18, 294–298.

Murray, C. & Lopez, A. (1996). *The Global Burden of Disease: a comprehensive assessment of mortality and disability from diseases, injuries and risk factors in 1990 and projected to 2020*. Cambridge: Harvard University Press.

National Institute for Health and Clinical Excellence. (2013). *Psychosis and Schizophrenia in Children and Young People: recognition and management*. London: NICE.

National Institute for Health and Clinical Excellence. (2005). *Violence: the short term management of disturbed/ violent behaviour in in-patient psychiatric settings and emergency departments*. London: NICE.

NHS Confederation Briefing. (2011). *Early Intervention in Psychosis Services*. London: NHS Confederation.

Pinfold, V., Smith, J. & Shiers, D. (2007). Audit of early intervention in psychosis service development in England. *Psychiatric Bulletin*, 31, 7–10.

Read, J., van Os, J., Morrison, A.P. & Ross, C. (2005). Childhood trauma, psychosis and schizophrenia: a literature review with theoretical and clinical implications. *Acta Psychiatr ica Scandinavica*, 112(5), 330–350.

Rethink. (2011). *Joint Working at the Interface: early intervention in psychosis and child and adolescent mental health services*. London: Rethink.

Rethink/National Institute for Mental Health in England. (2004). *The Early Psychosis Declaration*. London: Rethink.

Spencer, E., Birchwood, M. & McGovan, D. (2001). Management of first episode psychosis. *Advances in Psychiatric Treatment*, 7, 133–140.

Zubin, J. & Spring, B. (1977). Vulnerability: a new view of schizophrenia. *Journal of Abnormal Psychology*, 86(2), 103–126.

6

TREATMENT FOSTER CARE

Tim McDougall

Key points

- Treatment foster care has a relatively strong evidence base. Research from the US shows that it produces a reduction in symptoms and lowers rates of offending for mentally disordered and young offenders respectively compared to inpatient care or custody.
- Treatment foster care differs from standard foster care in several ways. This includes providing a detailed functional analysis and close monitoring of the child or young person's behaviour, providing substantial training and supervision for foster parents by case managers and by emphasising therapy. Treatment foster care services recruit, train, supervise and support foster carers, who usually look after only one fostered child for a period of 6 to 9 months.
- Multidimensional Treatment Foster Care in England (MTFCE) comprises prevention programmes for 3- to 6-year-olds and programmes for children (MTFC-C) and adolescents (MTFC-A). In addition the Youth Justice Board have piloted Intensive Fostering for young people in the youth justice system and the Keeping Foster and Kinship Parents Supported and Trained (KEEP) programme aims to prevent placement disruption, develop the parenting skills of foster and kinship carers and increase reunification and adoption rates.
- Guidance from the National Institute for Health and Care Excellence (2010) on the management and prevention of antisocial personality disorder suggests that multidimensional treatment foster care (MTFC) is an effective intervention for children at risk of going into care.
- Outcomes of MTFC compared with other care placements for adolescents demonstrate a number of factors that appear to lead to successful outcomes. These include good matching with the child and their foster carer; motivation and engagement by young people; early engagement of the child with their individual therapist and skills coach; commitment from the birth family, social worker and other agencies; stable school placements; and timely post-care plans.

Introduction

Nearly three-quarters of all looked after children in England live in foster care (Department for Education and Skills 2006; HM Government 2006; Department for Education 2010). These children have a five-fold risk of mental disorders, a six- to seven-fold increased risk of conduct disorder and a four- to five-fold increased risk of attempting suicide as adults (Meltzer et al. 2003; Department of Health 2011).

Treatment foster care, or therapeutic foster care, is a community-based multi-modal treatment programme. It was initially designed for boys with antisocial and offending behaviour but has now been adapted for use with girls. It differs from standard foster care in several ways. Unlike standard foster care, treatment foster care is underpinned by an individual functional analysis and close monitoring of the child or young person's behaviour, substantial training and supervision for foster parents by case managers and the provision of intensive therapeutic intervention.

Treatment foster care is based on the principles of social learning (Bandura 1977). Like functional family therapy, it draws on family systems theory and is part of a wider family of parent management training programmes which have evolved from behavioural treatment approaches in the US (Kazdin 2005) including the Incredible Years (Webster-Stratton 2001) and the Triple P Positive Parenting Programme (Sanders 1999). Treatment foster care services recruit, train, supervise and support foster families, who usually look after only one fostered child for a period of six to nine months. Substantial training and supervision for foster parents by case managers emphasising therapy is provided (McDougall et al. 2008).

MTFC

MTFC is the most widely researched example of treatment foster care and was developed in the Oregon Social Learning Center (OSLC) in 1983. MTFC has been shown to be a cost-effective alternative to residential treatment for children and young people with complex needs, severe emotional disturbance and offending behaviour. Children and young people in a range of US settings have been reported to benefit from MTFC. These include children who 'challenge' welfare services (Chamberlain et al. 1992); those in juvenile justice services with severe mental health problems and abuse histories (Leve et al. 2005); and children leaving psychiatric hospital care (Chamberlain & Reid 1991).

MTFC is listed in the US Registry of Evidence-based Programs and Practices and is one of the 'blueprints' that have been scientifically validated by the Centre for Study and Prevention of Violence in Colorado. It is recognised as a 'top tier' standard by the US-based Coalition for Evidence-based Policy. Only organisations that have received certification, accreditation or which are receiving consultation from TFC Consultants Inc. can describe their services as MTFC or use the acronyn MTFC. Standards for certification are agreed between OLSC, TFC and the Center for Research to Practice. A National Treatment Foster Care Implementation Team based in Manchester and London works closely with TFC Consultants and OSLC in a network partnership agreement. OSLC provides the National Implementation Team with consultancy, training and development materials. In turn the National Team provides these services and resources to local project teams, offering support on implementation, clinical consultation and support in adherence to the MTFC treatment model. As MTFC Network Partner, the National Implementation Team provides consultation to new teams wishing to develop the model for adolescents in the UK.

The evidence base for MTFC comes from several randomised controlled trials (RCTs), systematic reviews and other studies (Chamberlain & Reid 1998; Chamberlain et al. 2007; Macdonald & Turner 2009). Outcomes such as improved behaviour and reduced offending behaviour, for both mentally disordered and offending young people are significantly better for those who received MTFC than community, home or hospital care (Kurtz 2009). Positive outcomes seem to be dependent on four main factors:

1   the amount and type of supervision received by the young person;
2   consistency of carer discipline;
3   presence of a close confiding relationship with a trusted adult;
4   not being closely linked with delinquent or deviant peers.

What does MTFC comprise?

MTFC intervention during the foster placement and in the follow-up period includes four key elements (Chamberlain 2003):

1   provision of a consistent reinforcing environment in which young people are mentored and encouraged;
2   provision of a clear structure, with clearly specified boundaries to behaviour and specified consequences that can be delivered in a teaching-oriented manner;
3   close supervision of young people's activities and whereabouts at all times;
4   diversion from associations with antisocial peers and help to develop positive social skills that will help young people form relationships with more positive peers.

All children and young people have an individual treatment plan which focuses on problem behaviours and the development of skills for emotional regulation and conflict resolution.

MTFC emphasises clear and consistent limits with positive reinforcement for appropriate behaviour and consequences for negative behaviour. This is monitored and evaluated using a system of points and levels. Points are awarded for positive, cooperative and pro-social behaviours, and are deducted for negative or antisocial behaviours. Foster carers receive daily intensive support calls from trained clinicians in order to track progress against the treatment plan and to monitor their stress.

Children and young people who complete their individual programmes and move on to family-based placements are classed as 'graduates'. 'Early leavers' are those who leave the foster care placement within three months, and 'late leavers' are children and young people who stay in the MTFC programme for longer than 3 months but either don't complete the programme or move from MTFC to an alternative placement.

NICE guidance

Guidance from NICE (2010) on the management and prevention of antisocial personality disorder suggests that MTFC is an effective intervention for children at risk of going into care. The NICE guidance states that MTFC should be provided over a period of six months by a team of health and social care professionals able to provide case management, individual therapy and family therapy. This intervention should include:

- training foster care families in behaviour management and providing a supportive family environment;
- the opportunity for the young person to earn privileges (such as time on the computer and extra telephone time with friends) when engaging in positive living and social skills (for example, washing up and being polite) and good behaviour at school;
- individual problem-solving skills training for the young person;
- family therapy for the birth parents to provide a supportive environment for the young person to return to after treatment.

MTFCE

In 2006 the Government of the day published *Care Matters*, their strategy to transform the lives of children and young people in care (HM Government 2006). The report and action plan acknowledged that over a third of fostering services failed to meet national minimum standards on suitability to work with children and one in four failed to meet the standard on providing suitable carers. The report went on to suggest that high levels of placement instability and frequent breakdowns suggested that many children were not in the right placement or were not receiving sufficient support. Only half of local authority fostering services met standards for 'matching' children with foster carers. The strategy set out to increase the use of intensive foster care with multi-agency support, extend the use of specialist foster care for children with complex needs and improve the recruitment of foster carers through specially tailored recruitment campaigns (HM Government 2006).

The MTFCE programme was developed as a national pilot project in 2002 by what was then the Department for Education and Skills (DfES). By the time *Care Matters* was published four years later, nineteen projects were underway and the Government promised to launch new pilots to test the effectiveness of MTFC with much younger children and adolescents.

The MTFCE pilot was overseen by the National Implementation Team who provided training, support and consultancy and who, in conjunction with OSLC consultants, helped to ensure fidelity to the model of MTFC treatment. The first foster placements were made in 2004 and since then it has been developed at several sites in the country. MTFCE is the largest programme outside the US and the only national programme in Europe.

Rather than return children to families, which is the aim of MTFC in the US, the main aim of MTFCE is to provide children and young people with a stable foster care placement. MFTCE involves foster carers being supported by specialised clinicians to develop and deliver individualised programmes of care. These programmes last between

---

BOX 6.1   Core MTFC team

- programme supervisor;
- individual therapist;
- birth family therapist;
- skills worker;
- administrator;
- foster carer recruiter;
- education worker.

Source: Holmes et al. (2008).

---

six and twelve months and focus on empowering foster carers to bring about positive changes in the lives of the children and young people they are supporting.

There are three programmes aimed at young children aged between 3 and 6 (MTFC-P (prevention)); older children between 7 and 11 (MTFC-C); and adolescent teams for those aged 11 to 16 (MTFC-A). All programmes collect intake and discharge data and a national team analyses this to establish trends. The views of foster carers are also sought to help evaluate training, the experience of working with clinicians and applying the MTFC techniques. There is also a national research programme which is investigating variables such as parenting skills and competencies and stress levels amongst foster carers.

The Youth Justice Board have also used MTFC in a separate pilot programme called Intensive Fostering. This is aimed at young people in the youth justice system rather than the care system and the outcomes have been evaluated and reported (Biehal et al. 2010; 2011). Intensive Fostering was found to be more successful than custody in reducing reconviction, engaging with education and training and helping young people avoid antisocial peers. However, at one year follow-up some of the positive treatment gains made in Intensive Fostering were lost as young people received less support and gravitated back to negative peer groups (Biehal et al. 2010; 2011).

A typical MTFCE comprises professionals from health, social care and education services and is led by a programme manager (Holmes et al. 2008) (see Box 6.1).

MTFC-P

In a US study by Fisher et al. (2005) 90 foster children aged between three and six years old were randomly assigned to MTFC-P or regular foster care. Carers from both groups completed a daily report diary assessing children's attachment behaviours at three-month intervals over a two-year period. At each assessment point, the foster carers also completed standardised measures of the child's behaviour and their own well-being. Children who had participated in MTFC-P showed significant improvements in their attachment behaviours and placement stability in comparison to the control group. Foster carers also reported significant improvements in their stress levels at one-year assessment in comparison to regular foster carers. This was maintained at the two years follow-up. In comparison, the regular foster parents reported significant increases in their stress levels compared to what they were at the start of the study.

Children eligible for MTFC-P as part of MTFCE will be already in care and be aged between three and six years. Their needs and behaviour will have been assessed as being beyond the skills of regular foster carers and they may have experienced several foster or nursery school placement breakdowns. The aim of MTFC-P is to support children to manage their behaviour and to develop the skills needed to cope with and enjoy school. Standardised measures are used during the first assessment to help determine a baseline from which to monitor progress. Behaviour contingency systems are used to help children develop pro-social skills and behaviours. When children move on to more permanent care the foster carers support this transition to help ensure that treatment gains are not lost.

A 24/7 on-call service is provided and foster carers receive a daily telephone call from the MTFC-P clinical team. This is to help them complete the parent daily record (PDR) which tracks behaviours and foster carer stress. The foster parent also records information about the child's emotional and behavioural problems on a daily basis through use of a daily report card. This information is shared with the programme supervisor who monitors the child's progress and the suitability of the placement.

Whilst in MTFC-P the child attends a weekly therapeutic playgroup designed to support entry into school and success whilst at school. Activities promote social competence, emotion regulation and early literacy. The programme supervisor designs the individual treatment programme which is implemented by the foster parents. This is reviewed on a regular basis depending on the child's needs. Foster parents receive 20 hours of training prior to the child coming to their home. They then attend weekly meetings with other foster parents. In addition, a family therapist meets on a weekly basis with the child's biological parents to provide parent training and to address difficulties with parental management. This first takes place with just the parents, with the child being included after several sessions. Family therapy usually continues for an additional three months after the child is reunified with his or her family or is placed in a permanent home.

MTFC-C

MTFC-C takes a similar approach to that for young children. The skills that are focused on are those that support children to succeed in school and in their relationships with friends and the adults around them. In the same way as with MTFC-C, systems of behaviour contingency are used with older children.

MTFC-A

Fostering adolescents is no easy task. Research has shown that young people often reject help and struggle to commit to close relationships with carers (Stein 2009). Many troubled teenagers have experienced numerous, disrupted care placements and breakdowns in fostering. MTFC-A is the most common of the MTFCE programmes and has a strong evidence base for use with young people aged 11–16.

In a US study by Chamberlain and Reid (1998) 79 adolescent boys aged 12 to 17 with chronic histories of offending were randomly allocated to MTFC-A or a standard care control group. Their offending rates, school reports, out of care placement rates and self-reports from standardised measures were compared at programme entry and at one- and two-year follow-ups. The boys who engaged with MTFC-A were significantly less likely to be arrested or referred for offending behaviour. Their self-reports of criminal behaviour were also significantly lower than those in the alternative care group. In addition, adolescents in MTFC-A were more likely to remain in their placements and were less likely to run away.

Chamberlain and colleagues (2007) also investigated the outcomes of MTFC-A with girls. In a US study, 81 adolescent girls aged 13 to 17 with chronic histories of offending were randomised to MTFC-A and standard group care. The severity of the offending behaviour by girls in both groups was measured according to how long they were in custodial or secure settings. Self-reports of offending were also compared. Comparisons between the two groups were made two years after the girls began MTFC-A or alternative care. The girls who participated in MTFC-A were significantly less likely to be involved in offending behaviour than their peers who received group care. The MTFC-A girls were also more engaged in school and reported significantly fewer pregnancies.

In a Swedish study by Westermark et al. (2010) 35 boys and aged between 12 and 18 were randomly allocated to MTFC-A and treatment as usual. Over half of the young people in both arms of the study had experienced frequent breakdowns in their care placements. Parents completed standardised measures of their children's behaviour prior to starting MTFC-A and then again 24 months later. Both groups showed significant reductions in offending behaviour. However, the outcomes for MTFC-A young people were significantly greater than those in the treatment as usual group.

The two aims of MTFC-A as part of MTFCE are to help the young person live successfully with his or her family or another long term placement; and to provide the young person with effective parenting to support positive changes in his or her behaviour. To support these aims the young person's foster carers, parents or long term carers are trained and supported to provide the young person with consistent positive reinforcement, mentoring and encouragement to develop academic and life skills. They are also required to provide the young person with a daily structure which is based on clear expectations, behavioural limits and consequences. Supervision of the young person by the foster carer is an important part of helping the young person to replace negative peers with pro-social peers. Young people are required to take MTFC school cards to verify that they have attended school, participated and remained at school all day.

Drawing on individual and family therapies, these include those required to develop social relationships, resolve conflict and navigate the challenges of adolescence. Young people have weekly therapy sessions with individual therapists focusing on problem solving and positive behavioural change. Skills coaches support young people to develop social competencies and engage young people in positive recreational activities.

The Care Placements Evaluation (CaPE) (Department for Education 2012) comprised a RCT and a quasi-experimental observational study. The evaluation focused on two groups of adolescents – those who entered treatment foster care with the MTCE model;

and those in other care placements including foster and residential care. Outcomes focused on general adaptive functioning as well as mental health, behaviour, participation at school and placement at follow-up. Learning from a RCT of the MTFCE programme compared with other care placements (Department for Children, Schools and Families 2009) has demonstrated a number of factors that appear to lead to successful outcomes:

* good matching with the child and their foster carer;
* motivation and engagement by young people;
* early engagement of the child with their individual therapist and skills coach;
* commitment from the birth family, social worker and other agencies;
* stable school placement;
* timely post-care plan.

Outcomes from MTFC-A demonstrate reductions in offending, violence towards others, self-harm, sexual behaviour problems and absconding. Placement in mainstream or special school is increased and frequent non-school attendance is decreased. Behaviour difficulties in school are reduced (Department of Health 2006).

KEEP

In 2009 the MTFCE programme was expanded to accommodate the KEEP programme which is an evidence-based treatment programme originating from the OSLC (Chamberlain et al. 2008). This was to transfer the learning from the MTFCE pilots to a wider group of foster and kinship carers and children aged 5–12. The programme is based on the same theoretical principles of MTFC but without the whole team around the child approach. Lasting 4 months and delivered in 90-minute sessions, KEEP aims to prevent placement disruption, develop the parenting skills of foster and kinship carers and increase rates of family reunification and adoption.

Audit data from mixed groups of foster and kinship carers taking part in KEEP demonstrated significant improvements in behavioural problems, emotional well-being, and carer stress combined with significant improvements in parenting discipline style. Both kinship and mainstream foster carers report high levels of satisfaction and benefits for themselves and their children (Department for Education 2011).

As well as facilitating positive outcomes for children and carers, there is evidence that KEEP is cost-effective. The Department for Education estimates that each site costs £13,000 to set up which includes initial training, equipment and staff costs. In year one, running costs are between £2,500 and £3,000 per foster or kinship carer, on a four-month course plus follow up support groups for 8 months. The most significant cost–benefit is to placement stability. Estimates put the cost of moving a child to a new foster care placement at around £844, rising to £1,700 if the child is particularly hard to place. Cost savings are considerably higher if kinship placements are maintained, and higher again if the child does not enter residential care (Department for Education 2011).

Summary

MTFC is an evidence-based alternative to group or residential treatment, incarceration and hospitalisation for children and young people exhibiting antisocial behaviour, emotional disturbance and offending behaviour. Foster carers are recruited, trained and closely supervised to provide young people with treatment and intensive supervision at home, in school and in the community. MTFC has been shown to be both clinically as well as cost effective and is increasingly being developed across treatment sites in the UK and elsewhere.

References

Bandura, A. (1977). *Social Learning Theory*, New York: General Learning Press.

Biehal, N., Ellison, S., Sinclair, I., Randerson, C., Richards, A., Mallon, S., Kay, C., Green, J., Bonin, E. & Beecham, J. (2010). *Report on the Intensive Fostering Pilot Programme*, London: Youth Justice Board.

Biehal, N., Ellison, S. & Sinclair, I. (2011). Intensive Fostering: an independent evaluation of MTFC in an English setting, *Children and Youth Services Review*, 33, 2043–2049.

Chamberlain, P. (2003). The Oregon multidimensional treatment foster care model: features, outcomes, and progress in dissemination, *Cognitive and Behavioral Practice*, 10(4), 303–312.

Chamberlain, P. & Reid, J. B. (1998). Comparison of two community alternatives to incarceration for chronic juvenile offenders. *Journal of Consulting and Clinical Psychology*, 66, 624–633.

Chamberlain, P. & Reid, J. (1991). Using a specialised foster care community treatment model for children and adolescents leaving the state mental hospital. *Journal of Community Psychology*, 19(3), 266–276.

Chamberlain, P., Price, J., Leve, L. D., Laurent, H., Landsverk, J. A. & Reid, J. B. (2008). Prevention of behaviour problems for children in foster care: outcomes and mediation effects. *Prevention Science*, 9, 17–27.

Chamberlain, P., Leve, L. D. & DeGarmo, D. S. (2007). Multidimensional foster care for girls in the juvenile justice system: 2 year follow up of a randomized clinical trial. *Journal of Consulting and Clinical Psychology*, 75, 187–193.

Chamberlain, P., Moreland, S. & Reid, K. (1992). Enhanced services and stipends for foster parents: effects on retention rates and outcomes for children. *Child Welfare*, 5, 387–401.

Department for Children, Schools and Families. (2009). *Multi-dimensional Treatment Foster Care in England: annual project report 2009*. London: HMSO.

Department for Education. (2012). *The Care Placements Evaluation (CAPE) Evaluation of Multidimensional Treatment Foster Care for Adolescents (MTFC-A)*. London: HMSO.

Department for Education. (2011). Keeping foster and kinship parents supported. http://education.gov.uk/commissioning-toolkit/Content/PDF/Keeping%20Foster%20and%20Kinship%20Parents%20KEEP.pdf

Department for Education (2010). *Children Looked After by Local Authorities in England (including adoption and care leavers) – year ending 31 March 2010*, www.education.gov.uk/rsgateway/DB/SFR/s000960/index.shtm

Department for Education and Skills. (2006). *Children Looked After by Local Authorities – year ending 31 March 05, Volume 1: National Tables / National Statistics*, London: HMSO.

Department of Health. (2011). *No Health without Mental Health: a cross government mental health outcomes strategy for people of all ages*. London: HMSO.

Department of Health. (2006). *Promoting the Mental Health and Psychological Wellbeing of Children and Young People: report on implementation of standard 9 of the National Service Framework for Children, Young People and Maternity Services*. London: HMSO.

Fisher, P.A., Burraston, B. & Pears, K., (2005). The early intervention foster care program: Permanent placement outcomes from a randomized trial. *Child Maltreatment*, 10, 61–71.

HM Government. (2006). *Care Matters: transforming the lives of children and young people in care*. London: HMSO.

Holmes, L., Westlake, D. & Ward, H. (2008). *Calculating and Comparing the Costs of Multidimensional Treatment Foster Care, England (MTFCE): report to the Department for Children, Schools and Families*. Loughborough: Centre for Child and Family Research, Loughborough University.

Kazdin, A. (2005). *Parent Management Training*. New York: Oxford University Press.

Kurtz, Z. (2009). *The Evidence Base to Guide Development of Tier 4 CAMHS*. London: HMSO.

Leve, L. D., Chamberlain, P. & Reid, J. B. (2005). Intervention outcomes for girls referred from juvenile justice: Effects on delinquency. *Journal of Consulting and Clinical Psychology*, 73, 1181–1185.

Macdonald, G. & Turner, W. (2009). *Treatment Foster Care for Improving Outcomes in Children and Young People (Review),* The Cochrane Collaboration/Wiley, Chichester: http://onlinelibrary.wiley.com/doi/10.1002/14651858.CD005649.pub2/pdf/standard.

McDougall, T., Worrall-Davies, A., Hewson, L., Richardson, G. & Cotgrove, A. (2008). Tier 4 Child and Adolescent Mental Health Services: inpatient care, day services and alternatives: an overview of Tier 4 CAMHS provision in the UK. *Child and Adolescent Mental Health*, 13(4), 173–180.

NICE (2009). *Antisocial Personality Disorder; the NICE guideline on treatment, management and prevention*. London: National Institute for Health and Clinical Excellence.

Sanders, M. (1999). Triple P Positive Parenting Programme: towards an empirically validated multilevel parenting and family support strategy for the prevention of behaviour and emotional problems in children. *Clinical Child and Family Psychology Review*, 2(2), 71–90.

Stein, M. (2009). *Quality Matters in Children's Services: messages from research*. London: Jessica Kingsley.

Webster-Stratton, C. (2001). *Blueprints for Violence Prevention: the Incredible Years, parents, teacher and child training series*. Boulder, CO: Institute of Behavioural Science, University of Colorado.

Westermark, P. K., Hansson, K. & Olsson, M. (2010). Multi-dimensional treatment foster care (MTFC): results from an independent replication, *Journal of Family Therapy*, 33, 20–41.

7

MULTISYSTEMIC THERAPY

Tim McDougall

Key points

- Multisystemic therapy (MST) is an intensive family-based treatment that targets children and young people with severe behaviour problems or antisocial behaviour, including chronic or violent young offenders.
- The primary aims of MST are to reduce criminal activity, reduce antisocial behaviour such as substance misuse and violence, and decrease rates of incarceration, out of home placements and hospital admission.
- MST has also been studied as an alternative to inpatient admission for young people in psychiatric crisis. For a number of young people MST is not appropriate, but for some research suggests that the intervention may be more effective than hospital admission.
- MST is intensive and relatively expensive. Therapists provide a service 24 hours a day, 7 days a week for a case load of between four and six young people. Each treatment lasts 6 months and there is an average of 60 hours contact during the treatment period.
- The Department of Health has funded ten pilots across England to test efficacy. There are also existing programmes in other areas of the UK.

Introduction

MST has been used successfully for over 30 years with young people who are at risk of entering residential care or custody due to severe behaviour problems or antisocial behaviour. It is part of the USA 'family preservation' range of programmes and is recognised as effective by the California Evidence-Based Clearinghouse for Child Welfare and as a 'promising program' by the US Office of Justice Programs. There are currently over 500 licensed sites worldwide.

MST is an intensive, home- and family-based treatment intervention combining family and cognitive behavioural strategies with a range of other family support services. Its goals are to promote parents' ability to monitor and discipline their children and replace deviant peer relationships with pro-social friendships. Whilst MST is relatively expensive to provide, governments in North America and Europe have been concerned with reducing the long terms costs of antisocial behaviour and crime and have recognised the important 'invest to save' principles associated with these programmes. The potential benefits have been recognised by the Home Office and Youth Justice Board, where Intensive Supervision and Surveillance Programmes (ISSP) based on MST have been funded.

For services to be called MST or adaptations of MST they must be licensed as such by MST Services or their network partners. MST UK is responsible for ensuring that the MST model is followed by services using this model in the UK. This is because treatment fidelity and adherence has been linked to better outcomes (Schoenwald et al. 2003). The national team comprises the Department of Health, the Institute of Psychiatry and the South London and Maudsley (SLAM) NHS Foundation Trust.

What theory is MST based on?

The move away from treatment orientations that focus exclusively on the child has brought with it systemic and contextual explanations for childhood psychosocial disorders (Fonagy 2003). The conceptual framework that underpins MST is derived from social ecological and family systems theories of the 1970s (Minuchin 1974; Haley 1976; Bronfenbrenner 1979).

MST takes the position that the development and maintenance of antisocial behaviour by children is influenced by a range of individual, family and community-based factors. It is based on the premise that rather than provide individual treatment or family therapy, behavioural change is achieved through reorganisation of the young person's social environment.

MST developers identify nine key principles (see Box 7.1).

What does MST do?

The primary aims of MST are to reduce criminal activity; reduce antisocial behaviour such as violence and substance misuse; and decrease rates of imprisonment, out of home placements and hospital admission. MST has not been developed for intervention with young people who are living independently; those who are sex offenders in the absence of other antisocial behaviour; those who need stabilisation due to active suicidal, homicidal or psychotic behaviour; or those with autism.

A typical MST intervention lasts 4–6 months and the service is on call 24 hours a day, 7 days a week. Each MST therapist has a caseload of three to five young people and is expected to adapt their working pattern so they are available at times to suit young people or to respond to a crisis. Individual programmes are tailored to the needs of the young person. The family, peer group and school are involved in order to reduce barriers and promote generalisation of the interventions. Each problem area is individually targeted and action plans are generated. The young person and family are expected to achieve targets on a weekly or more frequent basis. MST aims to increase the skills and resources of the parents and carers to manage their young person's behaviours more effectively. Programmes are supervised by psychologists or psychiatrists.

BOX 7.1   Nine key principles of MST

Principle 1:   Finding the fit between identified problems and how they interact in the young person's environment.

Principle 2:   Focusing on strengths and positives as levers for positive change. By focusing on skills the family are already using the confidence of parents or carers can be developed and built upon.

Principle 3:   Increasing responsibility and decreasing irresponsible decisions or actions by family members.

Principle 4:   Concentrating on action focused and well defined interventions which help address immediate challenges and obstacles in a young person's life.

Principle 5:   Using targeting sequences to address sequences of behaviour that maintain the identified problems.

Principle 6:   Using developmentally appropriate interventions that reflect the young person's abilities and skills.

Principle 7:   Applying continuous effort through daily or weekly interventions.

Principle 8:   Using evaluation and accountability. The effectiveness of interventions is a continuous process. MST therapists are accountable for overcoming barriers to successful outcomes.

Principle 9:   Ensuring generalisation of outcomes so that parents or carers can maintain treatment gains when the MST programme has finished.

There are no MST specific therapy interventions. MST draws from an eclectic range of strategic and structural family therapy, parenting programmes, anger management and cognitive behavioural therapy. MST programme developers distinguish MST from other interventions by its comprehensive conceptualisation of clinical problems and the multifaceted nature of its interventions (Henggeler & Borduin 1995). MST therapists receive a high level of training and supervision and use approaches such as behavioural therapy, cognitive behavioural therapy and structured family therapy to support young people and their parents or carers.

What is the evidence base for MST?

Numerous randomised controlled trials, independent evaluations, benchmarking exercises and other studies have demonstrated the effectiveness of MST. The intervention has also been subject to a Cochrane systematic review where eight randomised controlled trials of MST conducted in the USA, Norway and Canada were selected and analysed. The Cochrane team found no evidence for MST over other interventions. However, this was due to the poor quality of the research evidence rather than the actual effectiveness of individual alternative services. The Cochrane team found significant heterogeneity among studies, small sample sizes and a lack of effects across studies (Littell et al. 2009).

A 14-year and 22-year follow up study by the USA-based Missouri Delinquency Project showed young people who received MST were significantly less likely to be rearrested or placed away from home in care or custody than their comparison group (Sawyer & Borduin 2011).

MST adaptations

MST has been adapted for some specific groups. These include children who have been abused or neglected (MST-CAN); those who engage in substance misuse (MST-SA); and young people with problem sexual behaviour (MST-PSB). MST-Psychiatric is an adaptation of MST that has been used to treat children and young people with serious mental disorders. MST has also been adapted for use with children who have chronic physical health conditions, but this adaptation is not covered in this chapter.

MST for child abuse and neglect

MST for child abuse and neglect (MST-CAN) is for children aged between 6 and 17 and has been used successfully in the UK, Europe and the US. It is an intensive therapy which provides a minimum of three sessions per week over a period of 6–9 months. It aims to address the multiple determinants of child abuse and neglect. The effectiveness of MST-CAN compared to behavioural parent training and group-based parent training and enhanced outpatient treatment include a reduction in anxiety, dissociation and post-traumatic stress disorder (PTSD); fewer out-of-home placements; and reductions in abuse and neglectful parenting (Brunk et al. 1987; Swenson et al. 2010). Current MST-CAN programmes in the UK include those in Greenwich and Cambridgeshire.

MST for substance abuse

MST for substance abuse (MST-SA) treats young people who are abusing drugs and alcohol. The evidence base derives from two randomised controlled trials (Henggeler et al. 1999; Henggeler et al. 2006).

In MST-SA young people are first supported to identify the underlying influences on their substance abuse. Following this an intervention programme to address and tackle these influences is developed. Drug and alcohol use is reviewed at each session. Protective factors which enable the young person to avoid substance misuse are explored and reinforced. Young people participate in training to enable them to refuse drugs or alcohol. An important part of MST-SA is random drug testing. Parents and carers are taught by MST therapists to identify and monitor young people's drug and alcohol use. Through a contract, negative results are linked to consequences and positive behaviour is rewarded through a system of incentives. There are MST-SA programmes in the UK at the Brandon Centre and in Cambridge.

MST for problem sexual behaviour

MST for problem sexual behaviour is aimed at young people aged 10 to 18 years who have committed a sexual offence or engaged in sexually harmful behaviour which has come to the attention of child protection services. The intervention takes place in the young person's home setting and with at least one identified caregiver. MST-PSB incorporates aspects of family therapy and parent training, cognitive behavioural therapy and social skills building.

The evidence for MST-PSB comes from three randomised controlled trials (Borduin et al. 1990, 2009; Letourneau et al. 2009). Lower rates of re-arrest and incarceration were found when MST was used compared to counselling or usual community services. Most MST-PSB programmes are in the USA but there are also sites in the Netherlands and UK including the Brandon Centre which is currently undertaking a research trial for teenagers engaging in problem sexual behaviour (Services for Teens Engaging in Problem Sexual Behaviour, STEPS-B).

MST with psychiatric supports

MST with Psychiatric Supports (MST-Psychiatric) is listed in the US National Registry of Evidence-based Programs and Practices (NREPP). Two randomised trials (Henggeler et al. 1999; Rowland et al. 2005) and one other quasi-experimental study (Stambaugh et al. 2007) have evaluated the effectiveness of MST compared to inpatient care or intensive community treatment. In one of the randomised trials MST-Psychiatric was found to be more effective than admitting young people with mental disorder to hospital for suicidal behaviour. Young people showed a significant reduction in rates of antisocial behaviour, had improved family relations, and spent more days in school and in the community (Heggeler et al. 1999).

The goal of MST-Psychiatric is to improve mental health symptoms and family relations while allowing young people to remain in school and at home rather than be admitted to hospital. MST therapists deliver treatment in the young person's home and work closely with parents and carers. Like MST more generally, therapists are in contact with the young person and their family on a daily basis, when needed, and on call 24 hours a day, 7 days a week. The average length of treatment is 6 months.

Because of the complexity of issues that therapists face, a full-time crisis case worker and a part-time psychiatrist are added to the MST-Psychiatric team. They undergo specialised safety training and are given skills to recognise and treat a young person's psychiatric problems.

MST UK

The MST UK national team holds the UK network partnership agreement with the MST programme developers and is responsible for MST sites across the UK. There are currently over twenty-five teams in England, Scotland and Northern Ireland, with several more teams being established following Department for Education funding for 'Intensive Intervention programmes for children in care and on the edge of care and custody'.

Although evidence from the USA suggests that MST is a very promising treatment the question of whether it is effective in the UK has not been fully investigated. A small number of UK studies have been completed by MST teams. Butler and colleagues (2011) evaluated whether MST was more effective than Youth Offending Team (YOT) management in reducing youth offending and out of home placements in a large, ethnically diverse, urban UK sample. The research team found that although young people receiving both MST and YOT interventions showed reduced rates of offending, MST reduced significantly further the likelihood of non-violent offending during an 18-month follow up period. In another UK study, Tighe et al. (2012) explored young people and parent experiences of MST using semi-structured interviews. Thematic analysis yielded a range of positive benefits for young people and their parents and carers.

The Systemic Therapy for At Risk Teens (START) programme was commissioned by the Department of Health and Department for Education and is currently underway in the UK. This has engaged 684 families across nine MST sites and seeks to evaluate whether MST is effective when compared to other interventions for young people at risk of requiring out of home care such as fostering, social care or custody due to antisocial behaviour. The trial is due to report in 2014.

Is MST cost-effective?

Based on a team comprising a supervisor and three or four therapists, MST costs between £7,000 and £9,000 per average intervention, and the operational cost of running an MST team is approximately £350,000 per year. The average per unit intervention cost is significantly lower than the average per unit yearly cost for mainstream foster care (£35,000) and residential care (£120,000–165,000) (Department for Education 2011).

Audit data from MST sites in England suggests that MST provides cost savings in terms of out of home placement, offending costs, police time and educational provision. Cary et al. (2012) evaluated whether MST was more cost-effective than statutory interventions that are currently available for young offenders in England. They found that MST reduced criminal activity and saved £2,290 per young person over two years of follow-up and reduced the need for youth justice services and saved £1,217 per young person over two years. They reported that MST cost £2,285 per young person but saved a total of £3,507, resulting in overall savings of £1,222 per young person over two years. These findings were consistent over time, and showed the same pattern of results when three-year data were analysed.

Summary

MST is an intensive, family-focused and community-based treatment programme for young people with violent, antisocial or offending behaviour. It is goal oriented and aims to help parents and carers manage challenging behaviours as effectively as possible. Numerous international programmes of MST have demonstrated effectiveness by reducing out of home placements, improving family functioning and reducing rates of reoffending. Programme fidelity is important in achieving maximum positive effects. Further research is required in order to focus on exploring which components of multi-component packages are effective and which young people benefit from which interventions.

References

Borduin, C., Schaeffer, C. & Heiblum, N. (2009). A randomized clinical trial of multisystemic therapy with juvenile sexual offenders: effects on youth social ecology and criminal activity. *Journal of Consulting and Clinical Psychology*, 77(10), 26–37.

Borduin, C., Henggeler, S., Blaske, D. & Stein, R. (1990). Multisystemic treatment of adolescent sexual offenders. *International Journal of Offender Therapy and Comparative Criminology*, 34(2), 105–113.

Bronfenbrenner, U. (1979). *The ecology of human development*. Cambridge, MA: Harvard University Press.

Brunk, M., Henggeler, S. W. & Whelan, J. P. (1987). A comparison of multisystemic therapy and parent training in the brief treatment of child abuse and neglect. *Journal of Consulting and Clinical Psychology*, 55, 311–318.

Butler, S., Baruch, G., Hickey, N. & Fonagy, P. (2011). A randomized controlled trial of multisystemic therapy and a statutory therapeutic intervention for young offenders. *Journal of the American Academy of Child and Adolescent Psychiatry*, 50(12), 1220–1235.

Cary, M., Butler, S., Baruch, G., Hickey, N. & Byford, S. (2012). Economic evaluation of multisystemic therapy for young people at risk for continuing criminal activity in the UK. *PLoS ONE*, 8(4): e61070. doi:10.1371/journal.pone.0061070.

Department for Education. (2011). *Prospectus: Delivering Intensive Interventions for Looked After Children and those on the Edge of Custody and their Families*. London: HMSO.

Fonagy, P. (2003). *A Review of the Outcomes of All Treatments of Psychiatric Disorder in Childhood: (MCH 17-33)*. London: HMSO.

Haley J. (1976). *Problem Solving Therapy*. San Francisco, CA: Jossey-Bass.

Henggeler, S., Rowland, M., Randall, J., Ward, D., Pickrel, S., Cunningham, P., Miller, S., Edwards, J., Zealberg, J., Hand, L. & Sandos, A. (1999). Home-based multi systemic therapy as an alternative to the hospitalisation of youths in psychiatric crisis: clinical outcomes. *Journal of the American Academy of Child and Adolescent Psychiatry,* 38(11), 1331–1339.

Henggeler, S. & Borduin, C. (1995). Multisystemic treatment of serious juvenile offenders and their families. In: Schwartz, I. & AuClaire, P. (eds). *Home-based Services for Troubled Children*. Lincoln,NE: University of Nebraska Press.

Henggeler, S. W., Pickrel, S. G. & Brondino, M. J. (1999). Multisystemic treatment of substance abusing and dependent delinquents: outcomes, treatment fidelity, and transportability. *Mental Health Services Research*, 1, 171–184.

Henggeler, S. W., Halliday-Boykins, C. A., Cunningham, P. B., Randall, J., Shapiro, S. B. & Chapman, J. E. (2006). Juvenile drug court: enhancing outcomes by integrating evidence-based treatments. *Journal of Consulting and Clinical Psychology*, 74, 42–54.

Letourneau, E., Henggeler, S., Borduin, C. & Schewe, P. (2009). Multisystemic therapy for juvenile sexual offenders: 1-year results from a randomized effectiveness trial. *Journal of Family Psychology*, 23(1), 89–102.

Littell, J., Popa, M. & Forsythe, B. (2009). Multi systemic therapy for social, emotional and behavioural problems in youth aged 10-17. *Cochrane Database of Systematic Reviews*. doi:10.1002/14651858.

Minuchin, S. (1974). *Families and Family Therapy*. Cambridge, MA: Harvard University Press.

Rowland, M., Halliday-Boykins, C., Henggeler, S., Cunningham, P., Lee, T., Krusei. M. & Shapiro, S. (2005). A randomised trial of multi systemic therapy with Hawaii's Felix class youth. *Journal of Emotional and Behavioral Disorders*, 13(1), 13–23.

Sawyer, A. & Borduin, C. (2011). Effects of multi systemic therapy through midlife: a 21.9 year follow up to a randomised clinical trial with serious and violent juvenile offenders. *Journal of Consulting and Clinical Psychology*, 79(5), 643–652.

Schoenwald, S., Sheidow, A., Letourneau, E. & Liao, J. (2003). Transportability of multi systemic therapy: evidence for multi level influences. *Mental Health Services Research*, 5, 223–239.

Stambaugh, L. F., Mustillo, S. A., Burns, B. J., Stephens, R. L., Baxter, B., Edwards, D. & DeKraai, M. (2007). Outcomes from wraparound and multisystemic therapy in a center for mental health services system-of-care demonstration site. *Journal of Emotional and Behavioral Disorders*, 15, 143–155.

Swenson, C. C., Schaeffer, C. M., Henggeler, S. W., Faldowski, R. & Mayhew, A. (2010). Multisystemic therapy for child abuse and neglect: a randomized effectiveness trial. *Journal of Family Psychology*, 24, 497–507.

Tighe, A., Pistrang, N., Casdagli, L., Baruch, G., & Butler, S. (2012). Multisystemic therapy for young offenders: Families' experiences of therapeutic processes and outcomes. *Journal of Family Psychology*, 26, 187–197.

8

HOME-BASED TREATMENT

Toby Biggins

Key points

- A range of CAMHS services are developing in the UK to bridge the gap between outpatient and inpatient/residential provision. These developments appear to be paralleling those that occurred in the US beginning 30 years ago.
- The range and complexity of these services makes them hard to understand, a process not aided by poorly defined typologies and limited consensus about service descriptions. Effective commissioning and delivery of these services and effective management of the service continuum is dependent on a thorough understanding of the different service types and their interrelationship.
- Evidence from the US suggests that more effective services share a number of characteristics including adherence to the CASSP principles, being targeted at specific clinical populations, being pragmatic, evidence-based, multi-modal and eco-systemic and maintaining small case loads with high supervision and a focus on model fidelity.
- New services challenge both existing clinical trainings and the existing service delivery infrastructure. Despite more than 10 years of significant service development in the UK, neither of these areas has significantly altered to take account of developments.
- There has been a reliance on importing US service models to the UK. After 10 years of developments there is now some considerable home-grown experience and expertise. Limited attention has been paid to the challenge of retaining this expertise and building on its foundation.

Introduction

Home-based treatment is a poorly defined term covering a range of disparate services, largely based on American service models. These services are designed to fill in the gap between outpatient care and residential provision including psychiatric units and children's homes. Services are linked by their intensity, their focus on hard to serve or poorly served populations, their targeted nature and their shared philosophical underpinnings. Using these parameters, the territory expands to include related family- and community-based endeavours, in addition to pure home-based endeavours.

This chapter sets out to bring some order to a muddled picture, beginning with an outline of US services – in part because their longer history has led to greater differentiation and a clustering of service types and partly because of an increasing focus on importing US services to a UK context, some of which are covered elsewhere in this book.

The UK picture is briefly covered. This neglect is in part because of the limited range of services, and partly because pragmatic and opportunistic service development has resulted in many having a weaker conceptual basis, although often US principles are evident. The author's own service is outlined, partly as an example of one model of intensive family-based treatment, and partly to illustrate a number of key issues in service development and delivery. The intention is to make clear both the differences between services and the common principles across services of this type.

The British context

By necessity, the description of US services is simplified, particularly to the extent that it implies a blueprint for an ordered, well differentiated approach to service delivery. In reality there are thousands of service providers driven by multiple and complex funding mechanisms with a geographical variability amounting to what one might refer to as 'rags and riches'. In contrast to the UK there is a comparative uniformity and changes in service delivery move relatively rapidly throughout the country. Nevertheless, a longer period of service development in the US has resulted in a clearer differentiation of service types than exists currently in the UK.

Until comparatively recently UK CAMHS provision was restricted to inpatient and outpatient services. While there was separate provision provided by social services and education departments, these were not related to or considered part of psychiatric provision. Over the past 15 years this picture has begun to change. On the one hand, existing services have begun to move towards more focused, evidence-based practice, and on the other, the range and nature of CAMHS services has expanded. Inpatient units have begun to move towards models of acute care with the place of planned treatment units increasingly under question. Acute inpatient admission is itself challenged by outreach type services. Concomitantly, CAMHS has begun to colonise its sister agencies with examples of mental health focused provision appearing in social care. Treatment foster care, Looked After Children teams, behaviour support teams and MST are a few example. More latterly, Tier 3 services, driven by the Choice and Partnership Approaches (CAPAs), have moved towards more efficient models of service delivery, the effects of which are only just becoming visible.

In the context of significant investment in CAMHS the driver for these changes has been in part politically driven, with a broadly defined inclusion agenda. However, changes have also reflected wider cultural issues including an increased focus on public sector accountability (with a push for efficient evidence-based services), a commitment to local and accessible services, a philosophy of patient focused care, and an increasing medicalisation or pathology and cure focus of areas historically considered from a more social perspective. To American readers all of these cultural levers will be recognisable, albeit they were predominant 30 years ago. Perhaps more surprisingly, at least for British readers, is the extent to which political factors also influenced the nature of service configuration in the US.

The US context

A review of the development of intensive services in the US is relevant to a UK audience for a number of reasons. Firstly, the UK appears to be travelling down a parallel road some 30 years later than their colleagues in the US. Secondly, many of the factors that drove US service development underpin British developments. The US provides a useful illustration of the range of service types that might begin to infill the territory between outpatient and inpatient services, and shows how such services, while targeted and distinct, nevertheless share a number of common characteristics. Finally, the US provides ample evidence of the dilemmas that emerge from more complex service delivery systems. By necessity the review is brief and no attempt is made to fully capture the complexity of 30 years of service evolution.

The US in the late 1970s and early 1980s was not very different from in the UK in the mid-1990s. Provision consisted of community hospitals, state hospitals, residential treatment centres and outpatient services. Large numbers of children were accommodated by the public welfare system and access to some services including residential treatment required parents to surrender their children into care.

Service change in the US was driven by two key factors: the increasing cost of provision and a rising concern about the numbers of young people in one form or other of institutional care. The publication of Jane Knitzer's (1982) *Unclaimed Children* acted as a key catalyst for policymakers. Knitzer described what she called the appalling lack of appropriate services for children with emotional and behavioural disorders. This seminal work galvanised federal action, resulting in the US Congress creating the Federal National Institute of Mental Health Child and Adolescent Service System Program (CASSP) initiative in 1984. Since their publication, the CASSP principles (National Institute of Mental Health 1983) have remained the clearest articulation of the philosophical position behind US public welfare and mental health policy. In recent years, similar principles have been evident in UK public policy. The principles required that publically funded services were satisfied a number of essential criteria (see Box 8.1).

In addition to outlining the underpinning values of services, the US federal government was interested in using clinically informed interventions to address a range of social difficulties including family breakdown, youth crime and substance misuse. This was again a parallel process that came to be observed in the UK beginning with the Department of Health's CAMHS Innovation Grants and progressing through to the development of UK-based treatment foster care and MST initiatives. The significant involvement of federal and subsequently state government in service development is not as surprising as it might at first seem. Firstly, the funding of the majority of US healthcare through insurance has inherent weaknesses when it comes to supporting service innovation, in particular

---

BOX 8.1 US Child and Adolescent Service System Program (CASSP) principles (1982)

Child-centered: Services meet the individual needs of the child, consider the child's family and community contexts, and are developmentally appropriate, strengths-based and child-specific.

Family-focused: Services recognise that the family is the primary support system for the child and participates as a full partner in all stages of the decision making and treatment planning process.

Community-based: Whenever possible, services are delivered in the child's home community, drawing on formal and informal resources to promote the child's successful participation in the community.

Multi-system: Services are planned in collaboration with all the child-serving systems involved in the child's life.

Culturally competent: Services recognise and respect the behaviour, ideas, attitudes, values, beliefs, customs, language, rituals, ceremonies and practices characteristic of the child's and family's ethnic group.

Least restrictive/least intrusive: Services take place in settings that are the most appropriate and natural for the child and family and are the least restrictive and intrusive available to meet the needs of the child and family.

---

in extending provision to non-core health areas. Secondly, the federal government has a substantial investment in healthcare via the Medicaid entitlement which is the means-tested health programme for individuals and families with low income and resources.

Of course, in many ways, the US context is quite different from the UK. In the US CAMHS is a far more fragmented system than the UK. At least six separate sectors or administrative structures may be involved in serving young people with mental health problems including specialty mental health; primary healthcare; child welfare; education; juvenile justice; and substance abuse (Stroul & Friedman 1986). Nevertheless an active clinical approach has always existed within each of these agencies in part reflecting the strong clinical training of master's level social workers. Historically, state hospitals played a significant role in the longer term psychiatric care of adolescents. Their closure through the late 1980s increased the pressure on traditional social welfare settings, such as residential treatment centres, to become part of the psychiatric continuum. Arguably, parents have been far more central to care in the US than in the UK. This is in lobbying for access to mental health services for their children and in securing a more collaborative stance from professionals. Such pressure has been supported by a less ambiguous view about the centrality of family life and a much reduced focus on adolescent autonomy.

By the end of the twentieth century, the service landscape was fundamentally different from 30 years previously. Some of these developments are summarised below. As the landscape has changed, debate has continued about the extent and nature of improvements, and increasing complexity has brought its own dilemmas. Some of these issues are discussed later in the chapter.

A service typology

Outlining a clear typology of the services that emerged during this period and that reflected the CASSP principles is a daunting task, not least because neither target populations nor service characteristics clearly differentiate the field. Indeed many common service descriptors – family-based; home-based; family preservation; intensive case management etc. – appear to be used interchangeably by different providers. Accepting this broad overlap, perhaps four typologies might begin to distinguish the field:

1 family preservation;
2 treatment foster care;
3 intensive case management and wraparound;
4 adult service model derived mobile crisis teams.

All four service typologies are multi-modal in the sense of delivering coordinated interventions that target multiple domains. Of the four service types, 'family preservation' is the most generic term since it encapsulates services focused on a child welfare population, youth justice population and more traditional psychiatric population. The uniting principle is intensive intervention in the family home with a significant focus on parenting. For ease of discussion below, the author has separated these three areas and chosen to focus only on child welfare services under the overarching model of 'family preservation'.

With the emergence of these services a broad continuum of provision can be identified stretching from outpatient through to inpatient provision (see Figure 8.1).

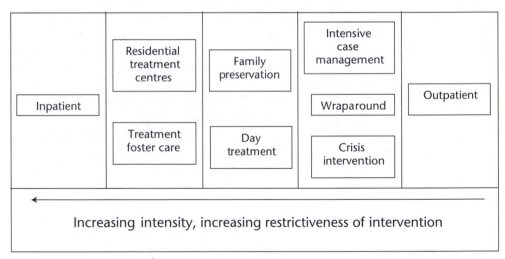

FIGURE 8.1 Continuum of service provision

Family preservation services

As noted above, 'family preservation' is partly a generic term, applied to many family focused, community-based services including MST. However, more specifically the term is applied to services that intervene with families whose children are on the 'edge of care' or to post-care reunification. The National Resource Centre for Family Centered Practice (1995) defines family preservation as comprehensive, short term, intensive home-based services for families designed to prevent the unnecessary out of home placement of children or to promote family reunification.

Family preservation has its roots in nineteenth century philanthropic child welfare. In the Children's Aid Society (1923) annual report it is declared that 'No child should be taken from his natural parents until everything possible has been done to build up the home into what an American home should be…every social agency should be a homebuilder not a homebreaker.' More recently, the Adoption Assistance and Child Welfare Act of 1980 (US Congress 1980) required US states to make 'reasonable efforts' to prevent children from entering foster care and to reunify children who were placed out of the home with their families. Family preservation services were listed as an essential component of demonstrating 'reasonable effort'. This was further strengthened by Family Preservation and Support Services Program Act (US Congress 1993) which is now called the Safe and Stable Families Program. Over the following decade these services developed almost universally throughout the US, although more recently the Adoption and Safe Families Act (US Congress 1997), with its emphasis on safety, permanency and adoption, has provided some counterbalance.

As with all intensive services, clearly differentiated typologies of services are difficult to identify. However, Nelson et al. (1990) provide a useful separation into services based on three models:

1 crisis;
2 home-based;
3 family treatment.

The US 'Homebuilders' programme is the best known example of a crisis model and is described more fully below. In Nelson et al.'s typology, home-based programmes focus on overall family functioning and their relationship to their community, providing both practical and therapeutic services over a longer period. Family treatment models focus less on concrete and support services and more on family therapy (see for example Lindblad-Goldberg et al. 1998).

In reality the diversity of services in this area is enormous but more intensive services do tend to have a number of features in common as defined by the National Family Preservation Network (2003) Intensive Family Preservation Protocol (see Box 8.2).

As in MST, the family preservation worker may deploy a wide range of interventions designed to provide broad-based parenting support; behaviour management training; family communication work; self-management skills; school interventions; concrete support; and advocacy, amongst others. The underlying philosophy is again strengths based, and whilst goal setting is collaborative some targets may be externally imposed by the child welfare system.

BOX 8.2 Common features of family preservation services

- immediate response within 24 hours;
- accessibility of staff 24 hours a day, 7 days a week;
- small caseloads (2 to 4 families);
- intensive interventions (8 to 10 hours per week as needed);
- service delivery in the family's home and community;
- usually short-term intervention (4 to 8 weeks), followed by other support services;
- 'hard' and 'soft' services delivered by the same worker;
- recognition of the importance of the interaction between families and communities, and help towards families forging those links;
- goal-oriented intervention with limited objectives;
- focus on teaching skills.

Source: National Family Preservation Network (2003).

BOX 8.3 'Homebuilders' core values

- safety is our first concern;
- it is best for children to be raised in their own families whenever possible;
- we are most effective when we work in partnership with families;
- people are doing the best they can;
- all people have the potential to change;
- we cannot tell which situations are amenable to change;
- a crisis is an opportunity for change;
- we are accountable to our clients and ourselves for service quality;
- it is important to reduce barriers to services.

The Homebuilders programme was developed by the Behavioural Sciences Institute (now the Institute for Family Development) in Washington State in 1974. In common with other services it articulates a core set of values (see Box 8.3).

Homebuilders shares both the service characteristics outlined by the National Family Preservation Network and the intervention components (Kinney et al. 1991).

Psychiatric family preservation services

The development of more psychiatrically focused family preservation services has lagged behind those focused on child welfare or juvenile justice populations. In part this reflects limited federal and state funding for development combined with the hurdles posed by insurance reimbursement for innovative or pilot services. One noteworthy exception is Yale Child Study Center's Intensive In-Home Child and Adolescent Psychiatric Service

(IICAPS) which was developed by Woolston and colleagues in 1998 (Woolston et al. 1998; Woolston 2007).

The service, which is now replicated by multiple providers throughout Connecticut, originated as a 'step-down' for inpatients but now also acts as a diversion from hospital and as an alternative for young people for whom traditional outpatient services are inadequate to appropriately maintain them in the community. In common with many of the services outline above, IICAPS is intensive, time limited, ecological and uses a phased intervention model. It focuses on factors that sustain pathological presentation or inhibit developmental progression while pragmatically applying evidence-based interventions to the symptomatic presentation. IICAPS deliberately targets engagement, develops collaborative care plans and uses a process of 'care review' (treatment plan refinement process) to highlight and problem solve treatment obstacles and limit ineffective treatment alliances.

Mobile crisis services

US mobile crisis teams are a publicly mandated and funded short-term intervention service designed to reduce emergency hospital admissions that are accessible via referral or directly by families. While access criteria and service characteristics vary across jurisdictions, intervention in all cases is limited. Typical services combine phone consultation and information with face-to-face crisis assessment, immediate crisis intervention and stabilisation and/or triage to an appropriate service including involuntary admission and follow up review or case management.

Treatment foster care services

Treatment foster care is now a comparatively well known service type in the UK, although it is generally associated with the Oregon Social Learning Center developed programme namely Multidimensional Treatment Foster Care (MTFC) and its preschool-aged version. In fact the UK has a much longer history in this area that can be traced back to the Kent Family Placement Project developed in 1975, and more recently the Coram Foundation's Fostering New Links Project set up in 1998 (see Hazel 1981; Brady et al. 2005). While neither service would claim to be clinically based both pioneered professional therapeutic foster care for adolescents who would otherwise have been served in residential care. The first clinically focused treatment foster care service in the UK was the ROSTA Project. This was developed by the author and colleagues in Liverpool in 1998 as one of the Department of Health's CAMHS Innovation Grant Projects (see Biggins 2007; Kurtz and James 2002). While none of these services remain in existence, MTFC services are now widespread.

In the US the field of treatment foster care is significantly broader than generally known. The Foster Family Treatment Association, established in 1988, has over 400 foster care agencies in its membership. While MTFC services were developed for a juvenile justice population, the majority of services are focused on Looked After Children, reflecting the roots of treatment foster care as an alternative to residential care. More unusually, one of the larger providers, Mentor, developed a short term psychiatric treatment programme, using treatment foster care as an alternative to acute hospitalisation (Mikkelsen et al. 1993).

In essence, treatment foster care services aim to combine the best elements of foster care – a nurturing and therapeutic family environment – with the active and structured treatment of a residential treatment centre. Foster parents are regarded as professional members of the treatment team, receive enhanced payments via salaries or increased allowances, have extensive training and ongoing supervision, and work alongside therapists and other mental health professionals to provide a coordinated package of care. A fuller account of these services and local developments from them is outlined in Chapter 6.

Intensive case management and wraparound services

As in the UK, intensive case management (ICM) in the US has its origins in the adult system developing as a service coordination intervention in response to the closure of large psychiatric hospitals. In CAMHS, ICM remains the coordination and provision of services for individual children and their families who require services from multiple providers. ICM exists across a wide range of tiers but is generally applied to children with serious emotional and behavioural disturbance – a federally rather than diagnostically defined group.

The huge diversity of provision has hindered effective evaluation of these services. More promising studies point to a reduction in psychiatric hospitalisation and out of home placements. Many other studies report little or no impact on outcomes but demonstrate more effective coordination and utilisation of services and importantly high consumer satisfaction. One theme for note for UK practitioners is the fairly consistent evidence that clinician-led case management underperforms that provided by other professionals, although the reasons behind this are unclear.

Wraparound

While many forms of ICM exist, services can be broadly differentiated into individual and team case management approaches such as 'wraparound'. Case managers act as both brokers and providers of services, providing assessment, service planning, service implementation and coordination, monitoring, evaluation and advocacy, and in many cases holding a specific budget to underpin this provision. In some cases, case managers may provide direct clinical services including psychotherapy.

Wraparound is a team-based approach to ICM and is used in the majority of US states as the mechanism for achieving the federally mandated Systems of Care approach. Embedded in a theory of environmental ecology (Munger 1998) wraparound is a distinct form of ICM in that it reflects a clear philosophy of care operationalised via a well defined service planning process that places the family at the centre of treatment. Within wraparound, services and supports are individualised, build on strengths and must meet the needs of young people and their families across life domains in order to promote success, safety and permanence.

Wraparound services should reflect the preferences of families, and indeed they should be partners in their determination. Wraparound plans developed by the team, of which the family is a full member, generally include both formal and informal services and resources.

Ambitiously the wraparound philosophy includes an 'unconditional commitment to serve children and families'. Outcomes are expected to be measurable, predetermined and continually evaluated (Burns & Goldman 1999).

Juvenile justice services

The Department of Justice Office of Juvenile Justice and Delinquency Prevention lists over 200 model programmes, covering a range from early prevention to active offender management. However, the Surgeon General's Report on youth violence (US Department of Health and Human Services 2001) used evaluation studies to differentiate services into one of three categories:

1   model – demonstrates a high level of effectiveness;
2   promising – meets minimal standards of effectiveness;
3   does not work – consistent evidence of no effects or harmful effects.

They noted that few existing violence prevention and intervention programmes had met the qualifications of a model programme and that, further, the evaluations that had been done indicated that much of the money the US spent on youth violence prevention was spent on ineffective – sometimes even harmful – programmes and policies (Mendel 2000).

The Center for the Study and Prevention of Violence at the University of Colorado reviewed over 900 programmes and placed just nine in the 'model' category (Mihalic et al. 2004). These included MST, functional family therapy (FFT), MTFC and the nurse family partnership. All these programmes are now underway in the UK. A further 20 are placed in the less rigorous 'promising' category including brief strategic family therapy, the Triple P Positive Parenting Program, and the Strengthening Families Program for Parents and Youth 10-14.

Effective programmes tend to share a number of key features, in particular a focus on proximal causes of offending behaviour rather than more distal causes. Consistent with this, interventions are targeted at several areas:

1   reducing antisocial peer associations;
2   promoting parental supervision;
3   enhancing effective family communication;
4   improving problem solving skills.

The underlying frameworks can be simplified to reducing risk factors and promoting protective factors so that increasing educational attendance and performance might become a central goal of intervention. With the exception of some notable clinic-based services, there is a focus on multisystemic or eco-systemic intervention in the shape of intervening across multiple life domains.

With good reason MST is widely regarded as the most rigorous of the family preservation type juvenile justice programmes. MST is described in detail in Chapter 7. For the purposes of this chapter it is sufficient to note that almost all of the common service features outlined above are to be found in MST. MST presumes that multiple systems impact on a young person's offending behaviour and consequently the therapy or treatment is really a programme of interventions designed to impact on these influences. Assessment is closely tied to the model so that the MST analytical process includes an assessment of 'fit' between the identified problems and their broader systemic context. MST explicitly avoids labelling families as 'unmotivated' or 'untreatable' etc., placing the responsibility on the treatment team to overcome barriers.

Functional family therapy

FFT is an empirically grounded, family-based intervention. A major goal is to improve family communication and support whilst decreasing intense negativity. Other goals include helping family members adopt positive solutions to problems, and developing positive behaviour change and parenting strategies (Alexander & Parsons 1973; Sexton & Alexander 2002).

The inclusion of FFT in a chapter on intensive services might seem out of place since it involves an average of twelve sessions, usually clinic-based, that are spread over a 3–4 month period. However, in relation to 'style' FFT shares much in common with other services included in this chapter and is one of a range of 'imported' services currently being trialled in the UK. While MST pragmatically uses a range of 'borrowed' techniques to achieve its intervention goals, FFT is more clearly recognisable as a therapy. While MST provides a good illustration of how different areas are targeted, FFT illustrates how clear targeting occurs both within and across sessions. Its clinical model consists of five distinct phases (see Box 8.4).

Each phase clearly articulates specific goals, assessment foci, intervention techniques and relevant therapist skills. Over the course of therapy, the clinician will act to minimise hopelessness and low self-efficacy; interrupt negative interactions and blaming; build family members skills; model positive behaviour and create relapse prevention plans, amongst many other tasks (Alexander & Sexton 2002).

Less popular in the UK is multidimensional family therapy (MDFT) (Liddle 2005) which is a treatment for adolescent conduct and substance misuse problems. In common with FFT, MDFT is a phased treatment with a strong developmental focus that clearly articulates individual, family and wider ecological intervention goals.

BOX 8.4 Five phases of FFT

1 engagement;
2 motivation;
3 relational assessment;
4 behaviour change;
5 generalisation.

BOX 8.5   US Intensive programmes and their academic partners

- multisystemic therapy (Medical University of South Carolina);
- functional family therapy (University of Utah);
- multidimensional family therapy (University of Miami);
- 'Homebuilders' (Institute for Family development);
- Intensive In-Home Child and Adolescent Psychiatric Services (Yale Child Study Centre);
- multidimensional treatment foster care (Oregon Social Learning Center).

Development of services

From one perspective the development of services in the US has followed a similar path to the UK with providers pragmatically developing services in response to identified needs, service pressures and funding opportunities. Certainly the patchwork of services is best accounted for from this perspective. However, US academic departments, usually associated with large medical schools and university hospitals, have played a more active role in service development than in the UK. For example each of the well known models that have been described in this chapter is associated with an academic institution (see Box 8.5).

Many of these services are in effect laboratory developed services following a period of casual modelling research which involves identification of key aetiological factors or processes. They are often funded by federal grants either at the basic research or piloting phases. All have progressed to extensive replication by multiple providers in the US and in some cases internationally. Despite a number of criticisms including the ongoing involvement of developers via licensing; relatively small sample sizes; frequent failure to include 'intent to treat' patients; and the extension of these services to multiple populations, they are generally more reliably efficacious than alternative service examples provided by countless US providers. A number of factors are critical to this success:

- Casual modelling work has resulted in services that have clarity about which areas they target with interventions.
- Active piloting with the continued involvement of academics has resulted in both a refinement of the areas targeted and the interventions deployed.
- A strong focus on practitioner training has ensured not just that they have the requisite skills but also that there is stronger 'commonality of purpose' in teams and clinician hopefulness is more resilient.
- An emphasis on model fidelity not only supports service evolution via aiding the monitoring of service impact on specific groups, but also acts to inhibit 'therapeutic drift'.
- Active comparative outcome monitoring, in particular, against benchmarks acts to increase clinician performance.

Common service features

As alluded to above, the various intensive services have much in common, not least in broadly complying with the CASSP principles, something partly ensured by federal and state funding criteria. The services are targeted at specific populations and while some models have expanded their area of focus this has usually involved some service modification (viz. MST versus MST-CAN). While casual modelling has resulted in the more academically informed services clearly identifying in what areas they target interventions, this principle also holds more broadly.

Interventions tend to be both multi-modal and eco-systemic (Bronfenbrenner 1979). In other words they target both the individual and their family and their wider context. Few services are based on one theoretical model; rather they pragmatically apply evidence-based interventions as appropriate to the target area and to some extent the client's preference. While their focus on bio-psycho-social assessment does not seem a distinguishing feature from a CAMHS perspective, assessments tend to be closely tied to the intervention model. That is, they place particular emphasis on those areas identified as relevant by the service's change model.

Many services incorporate visual maps to summarise core assessment features and orientate clients, parents and clinicians to the intervention task. In all mental health work the neophyte clinician quickly learns that assessment is more than a fact finding mission but rather the beginning of an iterative process of engagement. Many of these services make this explicit, clearly constructing the assessment to both achieve and monitor the nature and level of engagement.

The focus on engagement remains a central feature throughout treatment, with many services having notable impacts on retention and service preference rates even where their outcomes fail to exceed service as usual. Assessments culminate in detailed care plans, characterised by measurable goals, which are regularly reviewed. While the process of assessment is, to a varying extent, manipulative – in that it guides families into certain areas and, when successful, inculcates families into the model's change theory – care planning is collaborative particularly when it relates to prioritising areas of intervention and identifying acceptable outcome goals. While some services simply proceed by sequentially addressing the families' outcome priorities, others employ a phased model with distinctly different intervention targets and goals in each phase.

As work progresses, services work towards small easily achievable goals. Philosophically, such services look to build on strengths, in line with CASSP, and give as much emphasis to building protective factors and naturalistic supports as addressing pathology. There is a focus on the 'here and now', and consistent with older family therapy approaches, aetiological factors are largely neglected on the basis that, where relevant, they will be manifest in the present. Many services describe work focused on overcoming barriers, an idea replicated in the author's service – described below – which uses the concept of 'roadblocks'. The reader might draw some parallels with the idea of therapy disrupting behaviours described in dialectical behaviour therapy (DBT). From another perspective 'barriers' work is simply interventions targeted at relevant aetiological factors.

The emphasis on the 'here and now' lends itself to an action orientated approach, which is at the core of all intensive services. MST places emphasis on both within session and between session 'effort' by treatment participants. While few, if any, services so clearly articulate this idea, it would no doubt resonate with all as a goal of their endeavours.

Family focused services

A key driver for the development of CASSP was the recognition that the parents of young people with serious emotional and behavioural disorders were often inappropriately marginalised and pathologised. There is evidence that a supportive, non-blaming approach can help gain a degree of acceptance among parents (Ghate & Ramella 2002). Intensive community and home-based services place family at their heart and, more specifically, parental empowerment. Services explicitly ally with parental hierarchy and work to place parents and their children at the centre of the service delivery system. When this relationship is mediated, as it is in intensive case management, it is noteworthy that clinical mediators or case managers prove significantly less effective than more 'lay' mediators.

Across such a wide array of services one might expect the intensity of provision to be highly varied. Whilst of course variation occurs, there is an unexpected level of consistency. Caseloads vary little from a range of five to ten families per practitioner and few interventions persist longer than 6 months with many of much shorter duration. While all services involve some degree of weaning towards the end of treatment, in contrast to crisis services, intervention levels remain relatively consistent throughout treatment although the priorities or focus of intervention may shift. Access to clinicians is high across intensive services with most providing 24/365 access to the key worker rather than to a team member on a rota. In part to protect staff members from inappropriate workloads and in part to temper dependency issues, the role of the key worker outside of sessions is usually circumscribed.

While the better known services are manualised and consequently emphasise model fidelity, almost all services operate a parallel process that is designed to monitor and minimise therapeutic drift. In replication services in the UK, notably MST and treatment foster care, some clinicians have struggled with the impact of this on their sense of clinician autonomy. Nevertheless, there is clear evidence from the US that intensive services are particularly vulnerable to 'drift' and that, when his occurs, outcomes are negatively impacted.

High supervision levels are a consistent feature of intensive services. In some cases minimum levels are prescribed by state funding bodies. Daily plus contact is not unusual and supervision often proceeds according to a set format and frequently involves layers of supervision with the more distant supervisor emphasising model fidelity. For the best British exemplar of this model see the work of Bevington et al. (2012) on Adolescent Mentalisation Based Integrative Therapy (AMBIT). Finally, one cannot ignore the extent to which clinician style is both an important component of the effectiveness of services and also one explicitly prescribed by some service models.

Implications for inpatient provision

The development of such a broad range of intensive services over the last 30 years might be expected to have had a significant impact on inpatient provision. However, quantifying such an impact is challenging. This is in part because national level data is not readily accessible and most published studies have looked at local level impacts, and because residential treatment centres have increasingly formed part of the psychiatric continuum and therefore complicate comparisons with the UK. Additionally, while most of the service types described above play a role in mainstream psychiatric provision, nevertheless the majority of their clients would not typically have received inpatient care.

Overall there is limited evidence that the demand for inpatient care has significantly lessened; however, there has been a marked reduction in lengths of stay. Whilst a number of factors are likely to have impacted on this, not least the advent of managed care, an increased availability of intensive community services is likely to have played a role. Writing in the Archives of General Psychiatry, Case et al. (2007) report a 63 per cent decline in length of stay between 1990 and 2000 with the average falling from 12.2 days to 4.5 days. Studies of residential care also indicate significant reductions in lengths of stay, for example following the introduction of the Milwaukee psychiatrically focused wraparound service, residential lengths of stay decreased from 14 months to 3.5 months.

Up to date information on UK inpatient lengths of stay is not readily available and it is likely that there has been a reduction since the publication of the National Inpatient Child and Adolescent Psychiatry Study (NICAPS) survey in 1999, when the mean reported length of stay was 3.7 months (O'Herlihy et al. 1999). Nevertheless, there is a significant discrepancy between lengths of stay in the UK and the US. The comparatively recent tendency to separate acute and planned treatment units combined with the development of Tier 4 outreach and crisis services and some other intensive community services is likely to narrow this margin over time.

The impact of service developments

It is not possible within the constraints of this chapter to summarise the evidence base for such a broad range of services. Some are covered elsewhere in this book, and the interested reader is referred to the National Registry of Evidence-based Programs and Practices provided by Substance Abuse and Mental Health Services Administration (SAMHSA). What is clear from the evidence is that no one of the new service types can claim to significantly outperform the others. Examples exist within each type of services that have, with a degree of rigour, demonstrated both improved outcomes and client satisfaction.

There is strong evidence that the effective services are those that have strong conceptual models, high degrees of programme oversight and a focus on model fidelity. While it might be argued that this is simply a product of academically developed services having the resources to demonstrate effectiveness, this argument is countered by state sponsored comparative service evaluations that have reached similar conclusions. However, reasonably, one would expect that some highly effective services exist for which there is little published evidence.

Over the past 30 years the children's mental health and social care system has evolved from a fairly simple one comprising a limited number of services to a highly complex system with multiple service types and multiple examples of each type. From a purchaser's perspective this has presented challenges. In particular this has been in the areas of quality assurance, access thresholds and care pathways. While 30 years ago it would have been relatively easy to apply the UK mental health tiers to the US, today this would be an impossible task. The various intensive service types are not easily differentiated on the grounds of functioning or severity of presentation and each type may operate across multiple levels as, indeed, might single services. State funding agencies continue to grapple with this issue; a task not helped by the very broad definition of serious emotional and behavioural disorders.

The development of these services has involved a diminution of the specific care role both in mental health and social welfare services. Workers are increasingly expected to be sophisticated technicians. As the service review outlined above indicates, treatment models require their staff to be proficient in a wide range of evidence-based interventions. Equally, these new job roles require a degree of flexibility and working conditions that are not immediately appealing to more qualified professionals.

Each of the effective services, whether this is MST or treatment foster care, have required years of development and ongoing refinement before being able to consistently demonstrate effective outcomes. For professionals working directly in these services there is generally a comparatively short 'shelf life'. In the UK both imported manualised replication services and local initiatives have been made highly vulnerable by the loss of senior staff. In the US the involvement of large academic mental health providers and, effectively, a system of franchising has helped to maintain both developers and experienced senior staff members with services over the long term. However, even in the US, the number of such centres is limited which, perhaps in part, accounts for the proliferation of service examples and the variability of service quality.

UK service developments

Whilst in the UK changes in the configuration of services have lagged behind the US and been different in extent, similar changes have and continue to occur. Any reader of government health and social policy over the past 10 years would recognise at least similar sentiments to the CASSP principles. The continued drive for joined up practice and multi-agency working bears many similarities to the US Systems of Care philosophy.

The past 15 years has seen a significant increase in public investment in CAMHS services and, as in the US, there has been a clear bias towards social welfare issues and underserved or marginalised populations. The presence of CAMHS professionals in traditionally social care, education and youth justice settings is markedly different than in the mid-1990s and concomitantly a far greater range of interventions are clinically informed. Nowhere is this more evident than in the area of antisocial behaviour and parenting. The previous government's Social Exclusion Unit set the political context for many of the US evidence-based programmes to be imported to the UK but this was disbanded in 2010.

US residential treatment centers (RTCs), which are in effect large children's homes with on-site education and mental health services, have never existed in the UK. However, their precursors, 'Children's Villages' such as 'Boys Town' were pioneered in the UK, and some larger residential schools bear some resemblance to RTCs. Nevertheless, UK children's homes have not transitioned into being, in effect, longer stay hospital settings as many did in the US.

With the exception of RTCs, most other US intensive services have some equivalence in the UK. In the area of youth justice there has been a significant investment in prevention programmes with a particular focus on parenting interventions. MST, FFT and multidimensional treatment foster care are all currently operating in the UK under licence from their developers. Aspects of intensive case management are recognisable in the 'team around the child' (TAC), 'team around the family' (TAF) concept and 'child in need' (CIN) process. However, none has really attempted or achieved the centrality of the family that wraparound delivers. In adult services, personal health budgets have resulted in similar empowerment of the client but without the support of a well delineated planning process.

Whilst the development of services in the UK has been driven by government policy initiatives and related funding opportunities, there has not been the same level of involvement by academic departments whose role has generally been restricted to evaluation studies. Services have tended to be either imported, mostly from the US, or have been developed in an ad hoc manner by local NHS trusts and multi-agency partnerships. In the long term this approach runs the risk of fragmentation of services as exists in the US, with difficulties in determining their relative quality, and for sustaining imported services over time.

UK Tier 4 community services

Changes in child and adolescent psychiatric provision have come about more slowly than in many of the areas discussed above. Until comparatively recently provision had remained stable for many years although the underlying philosophy of inpatient units had evolved from a therapeutic community towards care in more focused treatment settings.

In the late 1990s, the first moves away from a purely bed-based provision was pioneered by Lesley Hewson and Ahmed Darwish through the Bradford home treatment service (BHTS) (Worrall-Davies & Kiernan 2005) and the community intensive therapy team (CITT) (Darwish et al. 2006). Located and operating differently, both services demonstrated significant reductions in both admission rates and lengths of stay.

BHTS

The BHTS focused exclusively on adolescents and was a 'virtual' team drawn from Tier 3 clinicians, although subsequently more dedicated community psychiatric nurse (CPN) time was added when it was 'overlapped' with an early intervention in psychosis service. BHTS is harder to place in a US context since it combined elements of various service types including mobile crisis teams, intensive case management and more psychiatrically focused wraparound services. The service had a stronger, but by no means exclusive, focus on psychosis than CITT and provided rapid assessment and crisis intervention, followed by 7–10 days of intensive support before titrating intervention as its case management function began to draw on Tier 3 and multi-agency resources.

CITT

The CITT bears some resemblance to Yale's IICAPS described above. As a free-standing Tier 4 team, CITT provided services to 5- to 18-year-olds with approximately one third presenting with emotional or eating disorders and another third with conduct difficulties. The service combined a strong focus on engagement, with containment focused and eco-systemic interventions. This was alongside high intensity supportive therapy and motivational work, and lower intensity 'high tech' psychotherapeutic interventions. The average client received 40 sessions from the CITT.

Over the past 5 years there has been a rapid escalation in the pace of change with new intensive community services developing throughout the UK. Indeed, we appear to be moving towards a position where nearly all areas will have a service of one form or another. Making sense of these new developments is a daunting task, not least in their labels that include teams described, amongst others, as:

- crisis;
- intensive outreach;
- assertive outreach;
- community outreach;
- crisis resolution and home treatment;
- intensive home treatment.

In common with the US, these labels provide little help in differentiating their focus or activity. In searching for a typological framework, one might, tentatively differentiate four service types:

a   *Tier 3 alternatives:* Services working with young people whose risk and level of functioning is appropriate for care within Tier 3 but who, for various reasons, are hard to serve and therefore benefit from more flexible provision. Such services usually place a significant focus on engagement, motivational interviewing and the brokering of non-traditional interventions – for example, Bexley's Assertive Outreach service.

b   *Tier 4 diversions:* Services whose primary goal is to divert young people from emergency inpatient admission. In common with the Bradford service, there is a focus on rapid response, crisis intervention and interventions that are usually both brief and loaded towards the 'front end' of treatment with the subsequent brokering of follow up services – for example Shropshire's 'Reaching Out' service.

c   *Tier 4 alternatives:* Services whose primary goal is to provide an equivalent treatment, involving a similar combination of interventions for a similar duration, to that received on an inpatient unit. Such services often recruit families as co-therapists in the treatment process – for example Cheshire and Merseyside's home-based therapy service (described below) and Solihull's Intensive Community Outreach Service (ICOS) as reported by Smyth and Hoult (2000).

d   *'Do it all' services:* Services that attempt to accomplish all of the above and sometimes more. Such services typically combine rapid crisis intervention, intensive home-based intervention, and outreach work with hard to serve young people – for example Wakefield's Crisis Team.

Service delivery and commissioning issues

Anyone who has developed or provided one of the intensive services outlined so far will be familiar with the enormous range of obstacles that inhibit successful service delivery. It is only possible to highlight a small number of issues that have emerged consistently across a range of services.

Difficulties often begin at the commissioning stage with poorly defined and or competing agendas that are particularly pronounced in multi-agency initiatives. Commissioners have often failed to fully understand the populations for whom they are commissioning services, or the treatment methodologies associated with them. A frustration with the complexity of clients has often been expressed via poorly founded criticism of existing services, and a naivety about how their needs might be best met. Equally, there has been a strong focus on establishing services with limited attention paid to the nature and efficacy of interventions and the complexity involved in developing and delivering new ones. As MST and its related services demonstrate, the process of effective service development is prolonged and involves considerable refinement over time. Many UK services have developed in an unstable commissioning environment with unrealistic short-term outcome goals, timescales and funding commitments that rarely extend beyond two years.

Most of the more successful US services have had clearly defined target populations with significant underlying work being conducted to identify their homeogenic and heterogenic features. Partly for commissioning reasons, UK services have often been expected to meet the needs of very disparate groups of young people with unifying characteristics not extending beyond terms such as 'complex', 'hard to reach' or 'hard to serve'. As in the US, care pathways have been poorly developed in CAMHS and related services. Whilst this situation is improving, the deficit has posed challenges in clearly locating new services in a system of care and consequently agreeing and managing access thresholds.

The 'continuum of care' model in the US replaces the more traditional model of outpatient and inpatient services with intermediate levels of locally based intensive care, such as home-based treatments (Bickman et al. 1995). Issues related to the location of services extend beyond where they fit in a continuum of care to debates about service boundaries. A tension has existed between integrating or co-locating services or establishing them in a more 'free-standing' manner. Many early UK developments were charged not only with delivering innovative practice, but also changing the culture of the wider delivery system (see in particular the CAMHS Innovation Projects (Kurtz & James 2002). Project leads, faced with the task of 'shifting' staff members' practice have often favoured strong service boundaries but have subsequently had to grapple with issues raised by service isolation.

Aside from the licensed service models from the US, on coming into being many teams have had to commence the task of developing an intervention model (what they will do and how they will do it) whilst simultaneously facing immediate delivery expectations. Solutions have been varied but have tended to cluster around:

- practice as usual in a different setting (some of the outreach services would fall into this category);
- targeted and coordinated intervention but without a clear conceptual model (Bradford's Home Treatment service might fit here);
- conceptually based or 'modelled' services (for example, Islington's Adolescent Outreach Service based on AMBIT.

In the US there was often a significant time delay between the development of new services and professional trainings taking account of them. This is a situation that remains only partially rectified. In the UK professionals taking up post often find themselves with no experience and limited knowledge about the service types they are tasked with providing. For service leads these pressures are particularly pronounced. Imported services have been able to partially ameliorate these issues by high levels of contact, usually weekly, with experienced service practitioners.

Staffing issues have been one of the major challenges for new services. Staff members are expected to have basic competencies in a very broad range of interventions, and are also expected to work unsocial hours, provide an on-call service and spend a large amount of time travelling to work. This is in challenging environments and whilst managing high degrees of risk and anxiety. The short-term nature of funding can bring a sense of job insecurity, and it follows that many services have struggled with staff retention. For 'imported' services there have also been cultural challenges. US services are typically far more hierarchical in style than is in the norm in the UK and the perceived loss of clinician autonomy required by model fidelity has gone against the grain for many practitioners.

Faced with these somewhat overwhelming hurdles the proliferation of new and innovative CAMHS services over the past 10 years is a monumental achievement and a credit to the determination of many of those involved. Looking ahead, the future for these service innovations seems uncertain. Politically there remains a focus on socially related programmes particularly in the area of families and antisocial behaviour as part of the 'Troubled Families' agenda. At central government level there remains a commitment to evidence-based practice and an apparent preference for manualised and imported services, which is not by and large replicated at the local level.

Shrinking social care budgets, the incorporation of 16- to 19-year-olds into CAMHS and a more rapid 'throughput' framework in Tier 3 teams have each placed pressures on inpatient provision. At the same time there has been pressure on inpatient units to reduce lengths of stay and to increase their focus on the acute care model common across adult mental health services. Consumerism or patient empowerment is both increasing and politically supported. Evidence from the field of social care suggests that this can result in a shift away from traditional services. In combination these factors might be expected to lead to another decade of rigorous service development. However, constricting budgets and healthcare reform have further compounded issues already present in commissioning.

The last 10 years has clearly demonstrated that service developments flourish where there is a strong commissioner and provider commitment to development, and where these initiatives are nurtured over time. It remains to be seen whether or not the wider context will remain favourable for future innovation.

A case example: home-based therapy service

In the following section a brief outline of the author's home-based therapy service (HBTS) is provided as an illustration of some of the issues discussed above. HBTS is a 'zonally' commissioned Tier 4 service designed to act as an alternative to planned inpatient admissions for young people from Cheshire and Merseyside. The HBTS became operational in 2007 and in addition to intensive home-based treatment it provides consultation to Tier 3 teams and some limited specialist assessment. The team is led by a consultant family therapist (the author) and is staffed by two full-time psychologists, one senior therapist and two mental health workers, and operates on a budget of approximately £350,000 per annum. The HBTS accepts referrals from the 16 Tier 3 teams, five 16–19 teams and the three inpatient units in its territory.

The HBTS commissioning context was and remains complex. Like Tier 4 services elsewhere in the country, those in Cheshire and Merseyside Tier 4 services are brokered on behalf of local clinical commissioning groups (CCGs) on behalf of NHS England. Inevitably this introduces a tension between local, zonal and national agendas. From a specialised commissioning perspective the HBTS was developed in response to a long-standing commitment to expand both the capacity of Tier 4 provision and the range of young people served. It was designed to reduce Tier 4 expenditure, particularly on 'out of area' placements in the private sector. The Department of Health, who provided start up funding, regarded the HBTS as part of its strategy to expand emerging personality disorder services and wanted to build on the work undertaken by the ROSTA Project in this area.

Tier 3 teams hoped that the HBTS would resolve historical issues of access to Tier 4 services and concomitantly sought a solution for young people who who did not meet the criteria for inpatient admission criteria or responded poorly to that provision. Inevitably, the service has provided an imperfect solution to these competing agendas and the consequent tensions raised have to be continually managed.

In common with most other UK service developments, HBTS had neither the advantage of an academic department affiliation nor the advantage of implementing an imported manualised model. However, in contrast to many services, HBTS did benefit from the author's familiarity with and experience of similar US services and fairly extensive experience in service development work. This was as well as the previous experience of staff members from the former ROSTA Project where many of the ideas were trialled before being implemented in HBTS. In developing the service a degree of primitive causal modelling work was undertaken, particularly around defining the characteristics, aetiological factors and core change elements in what might euphemistically be called 'stuck' patients.

Starting with the basic framework of wraparound and family preservation work, alongside a review of relevant therapies and services including DBT, cognitive analytic therapy (CAT), FFT, MST and mentalisation, this causal modelling work was used to modify the basic HBTS service type. In looking at the relationship between individual symptoms or pathology and family relationships – or, more specifically, interactional sequences – ideas about 'social domains' as conceptualised by Hill et al. (2003) were used to organise therapy. Whilst the service began with a skeletal framework or model with which to organise its work, the intent was always to refine the model over time. However, as service leads will recognise, the reality of day-to-day provision severely limits the time available for such development opportunities and four years on the model remains largely unaltered and manualisation remains a distant aspiration.

The HBTS referral criteria are similar to those of an inpatient unit in terms of high risk and/or low functioning, but there is an increased focus on chronic difficulties. Treated patients can be differentiated into three broad groups:

1 young people with previous hospitalisations who have deteriorated following discharge;
2 young people who are in hospital and have had unusually long hospitalisations – typically accounted for by persistent risk and difficult parent/child relationships;
3 young people who have functioned at a very low level for long periods despite significant outpatient intervention.

Diagnostically, all young people present with complex co-morbidity with primary diagnoses being mood, anxiety or personality disorders. A small but significant number present with less common conditions, for example severe chronic fatigue and pervasive refusal syndrome, while in the region of a fifth of patients also present with an autistic spectrum disorder. More dynamically, young people and their parents often have a high degree of hopelessness, are overwhelmed and exhausted. They have often lost all belief in the capacity of professionals to help them, and family relationships are typically fraught or strained.

For treatment patients, the HBTS provides a fixed six-month treatment package including assessment that consists of three times weekly in-home psychotherapy (one individual, one parent, one family session), one to five symptom management and/ or psychosocial sessions plus on-call out of hours access to team members, usually the assigned clinician. Each clinician carries a caseload of three patients with mental health workers working across the team caseload. The service lead 'holds' the care plan with the patient and family in a similar role to the MST supervisor or programme supervisor in MTFC. The HBTS works with approximately eighteen young people per year in addition to its consultation and assessment activities.

HBTS treatment consists of a series of sequential phases each with distinct goals and tasks. The work begins with an initial meeting in which reframing is used to normalise the young person's and family's experience. The clinician acts to depersonalise perceived failures, to challenge the young person's and parental relationship to the symptoms and to place the loci of responsibility for change back with the young person and their parents or carers.

Assessment phase

The initial meeting is followed by the assessment phase which, in addition to undertaking a bio-psycho-social assessment biased to the model's conceptualisation, is used to impact on identified factors contributing to 'stuckness'. Assessment is prolonged – 12 sessions over four weeks – and is constructed in a manner designed to intervene on such factors as motivation, symptomatic understanding, self-efficacy, perspective and family member roles. Engagement is a core goal of this phase. The sequencing and manner of the assessment alongside a deliberately constructed therapist style are used to promote engagement.

Preparation for treatment phase

Assessment is followed by a preparation for treatment phase in which four weeks are spent planning the detail of treatment, preparing resources and problem solving obstacles, both practical and psychological. Any necessary risk management work is conducted at this point. Clinicians work to agree a 'suspend change' strategy with families in which safety is not achieved by a reduction in risk behaviours, for which symptomatic change is presumed to be necessary, but by a reasonable pragmatic response to risk that seeks to both minimise safety implications and to reduce the secondary impact of ongoing risk on family members. Increasingly the patient and family are assigned tasks out of sessions.

Whilst coping strategies are introduced in this phase and pragmatic solutions are sought to the secondary consequences of symptoms, the focus is not on change per se but the anticipation of change. Throughout treatment, the work is guided by a detailed, regularly reviewed and revised, care plan that outlines measurable goals and objectives. The focus of the plan is on the sequential patient and parent actions that are required to achieve the agreed outcome goals. The treatment process is overt and disagreements are openly discussed.

Symptom management

Treatment preparation is followed by two, four-week phases focused on symptom management. Treatment consists of the pragmatic application of relevant, evidence-based interventions such as cognitive behavioural therapy (CBT). The emphasis is on 'here and now' action orientated therapies and the stance of the therapist is one of a coach. In the initial four-week period the goal is for the young person to understand the interventions and to apply them on a daily basis with the parent working within a social domain framework to establish an effective support position. Explicitly, there is no expectation of patient benefit at this point.

Throughout this phase the clinician looks for intra-psychic and interpersonal 'roadblocks' to the symptom management work. Roadblocks are made overt, openly discussed, and both the young person and their family are given the responsibility to resolve or set aside these so that the work can continue. Roadblocks are not regarded as negative behaviours like 'therapy disrupting behaviours' in DBT, but rather their expression is regarded as a desirable and normal part of the therapeutic process. The goal throughout is on repeated, small and successful patient and parent self and relational actions.

In the second four-week phase, symptom management work continues with an increasing expectation of both patient benefit and either a reduction in the presentation of roadblocks or their resolution without clinician intervention.

In the final eight weeks, the clinician works with the family to re-establish family norms. This involves reducing the distortion caused by symptoms, increasing day to day functioning and to building long term normalised protective factors. The final four weeks of treatment is focused on helping families make sense of, and internalise, the treatment experience and to identify, and prepare for aftercare services.

Empowering parents

In common with other home-based models, the HBTS model allies with parental hierarchy although it respects the young person's autonomy in the area of symptomatic change. The service operates from a family empowerment perspective and works to place the family at the centre of the professional network. Attendance at professionals' meetings is avoided; instead the family is encouraged to convene and chair its own planning meetings. Clinicians may help families prepare for such meetings or may support them within them, but the goal is to avoid undermining parental responsibility and centrality. This position is quite distinct from a minimising of professional competence or expertise which the clinician confidently and explicitly conveys.

Supervision

The HBTS provides a high level of clinical supervision following a brief training in the clinical model. The service lead provides the clinicians' supervision, and they in turn provide case specific supervision for the mental health workers. For the first 6–12 months new staff receive three hours of phone supervision per week spread over six phone calls, and have 1.5 hours weekly face to face supervision in addition to formal case reviews. Supervision not only focuses on model fidelity but also allows for a detailed discussion of session content and for the planning of future sessions. Following this training period, phone supervision is reduced to 1.5 hours spread over three phone calls and face-to-face supervision is reduced to one hour per week.

In its development and delivery the HBTS has experienced most of the same issues as the other UK services outlined earlier. Its complex commissioning agenda has only been partly reconciled by the service's focus on the three groups of patients described and by the addition of consultation services for a broader group. It has attempted to resolve targeting issues by looking for commonalities in 'stuck' factors and differences in presenting problems in which different treatment technologies can be more easily applied without undermining model integrity. The HBTS has had an obvious but fortuitous advantage in the area of model development but has nevertheless struggled with refinement work. Despite employing well trained band 7 psychologists, its clinicians have struggled with the range of technical proficiency expected as well as with the softer psychotherapeutic skills and have required high levels of support. Staff members work three 11-hour days, participate in a 1:3 on-call system, spend up to 15 hours per week driving and work alone for the majority of the week in stressful environments. Inevitably staff retention has been an issue.

Outcomes

No formal research on the HBTS has been conducted and no external evaluations have been undertaken. However, the service completes CGAS (Shaffer et al. 1983), HoNOSCA (Gowers et al. 1999), Strengths and Difficulties Questionnaire (SDQ) (Goodman 1997), Family Assessment Device (FAD) and a relevant symptomatic scale for all young people on intake, at mid-treatment and on discharge. Additionally, patients, their parents and referrers complete a comprehensive service evaluation form following discharge. Results to date have been promising with 92 per cent of parents reporting that functioning is significantly improved over the course of treatment and 79 per cent reporting that symptoms are significantly improved. Parallel figures for young people are 66 per cent for functioning and 62 per cent for symptoms. In terms of measures, there is a 47 per cent improvement in CGAS scores (38, 56), and a 54 per cent improvement in HoNOSCA scores (28, 13). Similarly drop-out rates have been encouraging with 13 per cent refusing any treatment and 13 per cent failing to complete the planned treatment course.

Summary

Over the past 10–15 years, driven by many of the same issues, the UK has begun to mirror the service developments that occurred in the US beginning in the early 1980s. As in the US many of the services have already demonstrated positive results or are promising in that regard. Increasingly young people and their families can access both a range and an intensity of interventions without the need for restrictive or institutional care with all the disruption of family life, friendships and education that this may bring. While we remain some distance from true selective choice by patients and their parents in the services they receive, nevertheless, this fledgling continuum has opened up options that have never previously been available.

Culturally there has been a shift, and whilst we cannot yet claim to have truly family centred provision we have made huge strides in focusing services around the needs of young people and their families rather than professionals. Painful and disjointed as the process has often seemed, these service developments would not have occurred without the collective commitment of central government, commissioners, providers and a small number of dedicated and determined professionals.

The increasing complexity of provision has and will continue to bring new challenges, as the US experience has so amply illustrated. Inevitably different parts of the wider system have evolved at different paces, so that service success may hinge as much upon agreeing new working practices as upon meeting complex needs. Nevertheless we should be encouraged by the achievements. The approach of youth justice services has been revolutionised. Some of the most complex and disadvantaged young people in care now live in family environments with a concomitant increase in their life chances. Parenting support has moved from a poorly resourced sideshow to centre stage. In places the most troubled and abusive families are being given a real second chance that does not involve a naive acceptance of inappropriate behaviour. No longer does a minimal quality of life have to be simply a fact of life, and a revolving door of admissions is no longer the only solution to a crisis. The challenge ahead is indeed daunting.

References

Alexander, J. & Parsons, B. (1973). Short term behavioural intervention with delinquent families: impact on family process and recidivism. *Journal of Abnormal Psychology*, 81, 219–225.

Alexander, J. F. & Sexton, T. L. (2002). Functional family therapy: a model for treating high risk, acting out youth. In: Kaslow, F. (Ed). *Comprehensive Handbook of Psychotherapy: Integrative/eclectic v. 4* (pp. 111–132). New York: John Wiley & Sons, Inc.

Bevington, D., Fuggle, P., Fonagy, P., Target, M. & Asen, E. (2012). Adolescent Mentalization-Based Integrative Therapy (AMBIT): a new integrated approach to working with the most hard to reach adolescents with severe complex mental health needs. *Child and Adolescent Mental Health*, 18(1), 46–51.

Bickman, L., Guthrie, P. R., Foster, E. M., Lambert, E. W., Summerfelt, W. T., Breda C. S. & Heflinger, C. A. (1995). *Evaluating Managed Mental Health Services: The Fort Bragg Experiment*. New York: Springer.

Biggins, T. (2007). 7 years on: reflections on providing treatment foster care in the U.K. In: Yule, W. & Scott, S. (Eds). *Fostering, Adoption and Alternative Care Occasional Paper No. 26*. London: Association for Child and Adolescent Mental Health.

Brady, L., Harwin, J., Pugh, G., Scott, J. & Sinclair, R. (2005). *Specialist Fostering for Young People with Challenging Behaviour: Coram Family's fostering new links project*. London: Coram Family with Brunel University and National Children's Bureau.

Bronfenbrenner, U. (1979). *The Ecology of Human Development: Experiments by Nature and Design*. Cambridge, MA: Harvard University Press.

Burns, B. & Goldman, S. (1999). *Promising Practices in Wraparound for Children with Serious Emotional Disturbance and Their Families*. Vol. iv. Rockville, MD: Center for Mental Health Sciences. Child, Adolescent and Family Branch.

Case, B., Olfson M., Marcus, S. & Siegel, C. (2007). Trends in the inpatient mental health treatment of children and adolescents in U.S. community hospitals between 1990 and 2000. *Archives of General Psychiatry*, 64(1), 89–96.

Children's Aid Society. (1923). *Annual Report*. New York: Children's Aid Society.

Darwish, A., Salmon, G., Ahuja, A. & Steed, L. (2006). The community intensive therapy team: development and philosophy of a new service. *Clinical Child Psychology and Psychiatry*, 11(4), 591–605.

Ghate, D. & Ramella, M. (2002). *Positive Parenting: The national evaluation of the Youth Justice Board's parenting programme*. London: Youth Justice Board.

Goodman, R. (1997). The Strengths and Difficulties Questionnaire: a research note. *Journal of Child Psychology and Psychiatry*, 38, 581–586.

Gowers, S. G., Harrington, R.C., Whitton, A., et al. (1999) Brief scale for measuring the outcomes of emotional and behavioural disorders in children: Health of the Nation Outcome Scales for Children and Adolescents (HoNOSCA). *British Journal of Psychiatry*, 174, 413–416.

Hazel, N. (1981). *A Bridge to Independence: The Kent Family Placement Project*. Oxford: Blackwell Publishing.

Hill, J., Fonagy, P., Safier, E. & Sargent, J. (2003). The ecology of attachment in the family. *Family Process*, 42(2), 205–221.

Kinney, J., Haapala, D. & Booth, C. (1991). *Keeping Families Together: The Homebuilders Model*. Hawthorne, NY: Aldine de Gruyter.

Knitzer, J. (1982). *Unclaimed Children: The failure of public responsibility to children in need of mental health services*. Washington, DC: Children's Defense Fund.

Kurtz, Z. & James, C. (2002). *What's New?: Learning from the CAMHS Innovation Projects*. London: HMSO.

Liddle, H. (2005). *Multidimensional Family Therapy for Adolescent Substance Abuse*. Norton: New York.

Lindblad-Goldberg, M., Dore, M. & Stern, L. (1998). *Creating Competence from Chaos: A comprehensive guide to home-based services*. New York: Norton.

Mendel, R. A. (2000). *Less Hype, More Help: Reducing juvenile crime, what works – and what doesn't*. Washington, DC: American Youth Policy Forum.

Mihalic, S., Fagan, A., Irwin, K., Ballard, D. & Elliott, D. (2004). *Blueprints for Violence Prevention*. Boulder, CO: Center for the Study and Prevention of Violence University of Colorado, Boulder. Office of Juvenile Justice and Delinquency Prevention. Report July 2004.

Mikkelsen E. J., Bereika, G. M. & McKenzie, J. C. (1993) Short-term family-based residential treatment: an alternative to psychiatric hospitalization for children. *American* Journal of Orthopsychiatry, 63(1): 28–33.

Munger, R. L. (1998). *The Ecology of Troubled Children*. Cambridge, MA: Brookline Books.

National Family Preservation Network. (2003). Intensive Family Reunification Services Protocol. http://www.nfpn.org/Portals/0/Documents/ifrs_protocol.pdf

National Institute of Mental Health. (1983). *Program Announcement: Child and Adolescent Service System Program*. Rockville, MD: Office of State and Community Liaison, NIMH.

National Resource Center for Family Centered Practice. (1995). *Child Care, Family Services, and Family Support. The prevention report*. Iowa City, IA: National Resource Center for Family Centered Practice.

Nelson, K. E., Landsman, M. J. and Deutelbaum, W. (1990). Three models of family-centered placement prevention services. *Child Welfare*, 69, 3–21.

O'Herlihy, A., Worrall, A., Banerjee S., Jaffa, T., Mears, P., Brook, H., Scott, A., White, R., Nikolaou, V. & Lelliot, P. (1999). *National Inpatient Child and Adolescent Psychiatry Study (NICAPS). Initial report to the Department of Health*. London: Royal College of Psychiatrists' Research Unit.

Sexton, T. L., & Alexander, J. F. (2002). Functional family therapy: An empirically supported, family-based intervention model for at-risk adolescent and their families. In F. Kaslow (Ed.) *Comprehensive Handbook of Psychotherapy, Vol. II: Cognitive, Behavioral and Functional Approaches*. New York: Wiley.

Shaffer, D., Gould, M. & Brasic, J. (1983). A Children's Global Assessment Scale (CGAS). *Archives of General Psychiatry*, 40, 1228–1231.

Smyth, M. G. & Hoult, J. (2000). The home treatment enigma, *British Medical Journal*, 320(7230), 305–308.

Stroul, B. A. & Friedman, R. M. (1986). *A System of Care for Children and Youth with Severe Emotional Disturbances* (Rev. ed.). Washington, DC: Georgetown University Child Development Center, CASSP Technical Assistance Center Substance Abuse and Mental Health Services Administration, National Mental Health Information Center. Available at http://www.nrepp.samhsa.gov/Index.aspx

US Congress. (1980). Adoption Assistance and Child Welfare Act of 1980. Public Law 96-272, Ninety-Sixth Congress, H.R. 3434.

US Congress. (1993). Family Preservation and Support Services Program Act of 1993. P.L. 103–166, H.R. 2264.

US Congress. (1997). Adoption and Safe Families Act of 1997, P.L. 105–89, H.R. 897.

US Department of Health and Human Services. (2001). *Youth Violence: A report of the Surgeon General*. Rockville, MD: US Department of Health and Human Services; Centers for Disease Control and Prevention; National Center for Injury Prevention and Control; Substance Abuse and Mental Health Services Administration; Center for Mental Health Services; and National Institutes of Health, National Institute of Mental Health.

Woolston, J. L. (2007). *IICAPS, a Home-Based Psychiatric Treatment for Children & Adolescents*. New Haven, CT: Yale University Press.

Woolston, J. L., Berkowitz, S. J., Schaefer, M. C. & Adnopoz, J. A. (1998) Intensive, integrated in-home psychiatric services: the catalyst to enhancing out-patient intervention. *Child and Adolescent Psychiatric Clinics of North America*, 7, 615–633.

Worrall-Davies, A. & Kiernan, K. (2005). *Using a Virtual Team: an evaluation of the Bradford CAMHS intensive home treatment approach*. Leeds: University of Leeds.

9

FORENSIC INTERVENTIONS

Paul Mitchell

Key points

- Young people in forensic settings often have multiple complex needs and are likely to have serious mental health and social problems into adulthood if these needs remain unmet.
- Forensic CAMHS practice should embody the best principles of CAMHS practice (effective models of service delivery and evidence-based interventions) and forensic practice (robust risk assessment and risk management models), and should be benchmarked against standards for both.
- Interventions for other mental health problems should be offered in conjunction with interventions to address conduct disorder or high risk or offending behaviours. Evidence suggests that the most effective interventions for conduct disorder involve carers and the young person's support network through parenting and system wide interventions.
- Effective forensic CAMHS practice is based on robust case management and good inter-agency working, good information sharing, and strong engagement with service users, their families and carers.
- Forensic CAMHS is an area of practice and service delivery that is rapidly developing, and service models and interventions are likely to evolve further in the future.

Introduction

Adolescent offenders are known to have high levels of mental health problems when compared with other populations of young people. Studies in the UK (Chitsabesan et al. 2006; Kroll et al. 2002) and internationally (Teplin et al. 2002; Vreugdenhil et al. 2004) consistently identify higher levels of morbidity than among the general adolescent populations of the same countries (Costello et al. 1996; Meltzer et al. 2000). These high levels of morbidity are associated with poor outcomes into adulthood, including continuing mental health problems (Maughan & Kim-Cohen 2005), and further offending (Rutter et al. 1998).

For some time this population has been recognised as at risk for the development of antisocial personality disorder in adulthood (Bailey et al. 2007), but emerging evidence suggests that the prevalence is far higher than previously thought (Chitsabesan et al. 2012). Recent guidance (National Institute for Health and Clinical Excellence 2009) has prioritised early intervention for children in vulnerable families and at risk of developing conduct disorder as a key element of the strategy to reduce antisocial personality disorder in adulthood.

Apart from mental health needs, adolescent offenders also have high levels of other healthcare needs that impact on their emotional and psychological well-being. These include substance misuse problems (Hall 2000) and neuro-developmental problems such as learning difficulties (Kroll et al. 2002) and communication disorders (Bryan et al. 2007). Additionally, young people in contact with the justice system have higher levels of psychiatric co-morbidity (Abram et al. 2003; Vermeiren et al. 2006) and other areas of unmet social need, such as lack of access to education (Parke 2009) and accommodation (Youth Justice Board 2007).

Equivalence of access to mental health services has long been recognised as a priority within secure settings (HM Prison Service & NHS Executive 1999) and more generally (Department for Children, Schools and Families & Department of Health 2009; Department of Health 2004) for young people in contact with the justice system.

Forensic CAMHS: a stepped care approach

Although the level of mental health need among this population is high, the pathways and services they require are dependent on the nature and severity of the problems they are experiencing. Pathways for young people experiencing the early onset of serious mental illness within the justice system will not be the same as for those experiencing difficulties with anger control that may contribute to offending behaviour. In the first scenario admission to specialist inpatient provision may well be needed, but in the second case it is likely that the young person can be supported in their current setting. This has already been recognised and a 'stepped care' approach has been advocated in the commissioning and delivery of mental health services (Williams and Kerfoot 2005).

As with mental health needs, forensic behaviours vary in nature and severity, and therefore warrant different approaches to risk management and interventions. The most recently available figures for England and Wales (Youth Justice Board 2012) indicate that 21 per cent of proven offences by young people fell into the category of violence against the person. Although this is the largest single category it constitutes only one-fifth of overall offending. Therefore many young people who offend will not be referred to specialist forensic services, yet may still require support for unmet mental health needs. Therefore a 'stepped care' approach is also needed for this aspect of work, which necessitates a range of provision from generic to specialist mental health services.

Forensic CAMHS is a relatively new concept and is still being both conceptually and operationally defined (Withecombe & Jasti 2007). It consists of a combination of models and theories from both child and adolescent mental health and forensic mental health practice (Withecomb 2008). From a Tier 4 perspective it could be argued that only highly specialised services such as medium secure inpatient facilities and explicitly configured community forensic services meet these criteria, and that mental health services for adolescent offenders in other contexts should replicate the principles and service models of comprehensive CAMHS outlined earlier. However, this fails to take into account recent innovations in service delivery for this population (Hoare & Wilson 2010; Ryan & Mitchell 2011) that combine both CAMHS and forensic expertise, and also the interplay between mental health needs and risk that operates at all tiers of intervention with adolescent offenders. Therefore, although this chapter addresses the more explicit agenda of Tier 4 services, it also includes aspects of thinking and practice that are relevant to all mental health practitioners working with young offenders and those requiring similar services.

This chapter also explores issues several aspects of service provision, including assessment of needs and risk, pathways and service models, and emerging practice models. However, it is not possible to do full justice to these themes in the space available. A further limitation is that the chapter replicates a core problem in the provision of services to adolescent offenders in that it will concentrate on the needs of adolescent boys and make only brief reference to the needs of younger children, girls and young people from minority ethnic groups, all of which are known to differ from population norms (Lader et al. 2000; Meltzer et al. 2000). Again, this is unavoidable in the space available, but does at least highlight further the limitations of current models of service provision.

Context for service provision: needs, outcomes and access to services

Provision of mental health services for young people in contact with the justice system historically has been limited in scope and highly variable in character. In the UK growing concerns regarding short and long term outcomes for this group has resulted over recent years in increased provision at all tiers (i.e. from first level community interventions through to specialised secure inpatient services), but at a national level the access and availability of services remains uneven (Department of Health 2009; Khan 2010). A similar pattern is reported internationally (MacReady 2009).

An additional problem is that adolescent offenders are often reluctant to use services even when they are offered (Shelton 2004; Whittle et al. in press), which is unsurprising given some of the factors associated with service uptake in the general adolescent population. These include high academic attainment (Zwaanswijk et al. 2003), help-seeking for other problems (Gasquet et al. 1997), confiding in professionals such as teachers (Zimmer-Gembeck & Locke 2007), and parental or carer concern (Sayal et al. 2002). This raises the question as to whether or not current service models are fit for purpose. To put it another way, we may ask ourselves whether we are offering services that are correctly configured to maximise uptake by the target population. This will be explored further in the section on interventions.

Another important and related question is: what kind of services do adolescent offenders require based on what we know about their mental health needs? Clearly services should be comprehensive to meet all needs and be stepped in design in order to provide interventions that are proportionate to the young person's level of need. It has been recognised for some time that some young people have a combination of serious mental health problems and risky behaviours sufficient for them to require medium secure inpatient care. Historically this group has mostly comprised young people with serious mental illness or learning disability. However, there have always been some young people who have unusual or atypical profiles of need that were seen as complex and neuro-developmental in nature (although not always meeting criteria for a single diagnostic category such as Asperger's syndrome or attention deficit hyperactivity disorder (ADHD)).

As awareness grows regarding what are often complex neuro-developmental profiles among adolescent offenders, referrals to inpatient services for these young people are increasing. More and more the services to which they are referred are expected to provide appropriate interventions which are often psychosocial in nature. However, for many young people with needs in this area inpatient admission can be disproportionate, intrusive and unhelpful. As such, services in other settings such as community and the secure estate will increasingly be expected to provide appropriate interventions as part of a comprehensive CAMHS.

Hand in hand with the growing awareness of neuro-developmental problems comes an increasing understanding of the role that disrupted and/or multiple attachments and repeated exposure to traumatic events such as domestic violence and abuse, play in the presentation of young people in contact with the justice system (Office of the Children's Commissioner 2011). Such experiences negatively affect a child or young person's capacity for self-regulation and ability to engage in meaningful relationships with other people. For young people in secure settings this may manifest in how they engage with their immediate carers and professionals attempting to provide interventions. However, there is also emerging evidence that psychologically informed care delivered by immediate carers supported by skilled mental health professionals can significantly improve outcomes for these repeatedly traumatised young people, both in community settings (Henggeler et al. 1992) and in the secure estate (Ryan & Mitchell 2011).

Almost by definition young people in contact with the youth justice system will meet the criteria for conduct disorder, and this is particularly true for those who are placed in secure settings. This combined with the high prevalence rates for other mental health problems means that co-morbidity and, therefore, case complexity is increased, and the level of resources and expertise needed within services is correspondingly high.

Assessment of needs and risk

Comprehensive needs and risk assessment processes that inform case management are central to any service working with adolescent offenders, although the nature of the processes will vary depending on the context. Needs and risk assessment in a medium secure inpatient unit will by definition be more complex and detailed than those in a Youth Offending Service (YOS). However, in both cases the assessment processes need to be structured and draw on multiple information sources. The risk assessment should be dynamic (i.e. reviewed over time, rather than static or one-off) and inform clinical decision making (Mitchell 2006). It should also be part of a multidisciplinary and multi-agency case management process. Structured assessment tools are assuming increasing importance as outcome measures for several purposes. These include the evaluation of progress of individual service users, assessing the effectiveness of specific interventions, and evaluating the overall effectiveness and quality of services. Therefore incorporating structured assessment tools into clinical practice achieves several goals.

A structured assessment is one that considers multiple domains or constructs that are relevant to needs or risk in a systematic way. The domains are known to be relevant as they are evidence based and have some predictive value. A thorough assessment will draw on multiple sources of information, such as interview with the young person, information from carers or professionals, and relevant historical documents (Mitchell 2006). Multiple information sources ensure a more comprehensive picture is built up and permit separate pieces of evidence to be compared and weighted accordingly. An assessment drawing on one evidence source may focus on one area of need or risk at the expense of others and therefore potentially disregard important information. A dynamic assessment process is one that reassesses needs or risk on a regular basis or more frequently when new information is available or a significant change of circumstances occurs. The value of the assessment process is only realised when it informs clinical decisions regarding meeting needs or risk and it contributes to a wider planning process involving all agencies working with the young person. This issue is revisited later in the section on case management.

There are a range of need and risk assessment tools that are useful in the field of adolescent forensic mental health, some of which are described below. However, there are also omissions. In particular there is a need for a front-line global risk assessment which can be usefully applied in community settings.

Needs assessment

A number of needs assessments or screening tools have been developed and validated for use with adolescent offenders and they vary in their scope and method. The Salford Needs Assessment for Adolescents (SNASA) (Kroll et al. 1999) is a comprehensive assessment of needs (i.e. not just mental health needs) that uses multiple information sources to assist clinical decision making regarding the need for interventions. A more focused two stage mental health screening tool was developed from SNASA specifically for use within the youth justice system. This has now been incorporated into the Comprehensive Health Assessment Tool (CHAT) which is a multidimensional tool that assesses needs in five domains:

1   immediate needs;
2   physical health;
3   mental health;
4   substance misuse;
5   neuro-developmental needs.

The full version of CHAT is currently being evaluated, although most of the component parts have been validated (Bailey et al. 2008), and are already in use within the secure estate.

Internationally there is a range of tools in use, for instance the Massachusetts Youth Screening Instrument – second edition (MAYSI-2) (Grisso et al. 2001) which was developed in the US but is now used in a number of other countries. It is a 52-item self-report questionnaire that addresses several key areas of mental health need. The Basis RaadsOnderzoek (BARO) screening instrument (Doreleiers et al. 2011) was developed in the Netherlands and is available in several languages including English. It is a more general needs assessment that includes mental health and emotional needs within nine domains, and is designed to be administered by a youth justice worker.

The development and utilisation of assessment and screening tools has raised further questions regarding the optimal method and timing for screening (Bailey et al. 2006), given both the stress induced by contact with the justice system and the vulnerability of the population. The dilemma is between screening too early and obtaining an inaccurate picture distorted by limited information and contextual but possibly short term stress, and screening too late to identify risk issues needing an immediate response. It has been proposed (Mitchell & Shaw 2011) that a short term longitudinal approach may achieve the best balance between immediacy and accuracy, and current screening initiatives being developed within the UK combine an 'immediate needs' element at point of entry into the system with a more comprehensive subsequent screen.

More specialised tools may be used in relation to particular areas of mental health need, such as psychosis or ADHD. Use of such tools should be in accordance with current guidelines on clinical standards and best practice, but should take account of issues relating to case complexity, co-morbidity and risk management. Tools that have been used effectively within medium secure inpatient, secure estate and community settings include the Krawiecka, Goldberg and Vaughan (KGV) for psychosis (Krawiecka, Goldberg & Vaughan 1977), Connors for ADHD (Conners et al. 1998) and Trauma Symptom Checklist (Briere 1996) for trauma.

Risk assessment

Risk assessment tools validated with adolescent offenders tend to focus on a specific area of risk rather than being global in nature, and usually require specific training prior to use. As with needs assessment tools, they have utility in informing clinical decision making and also in assessing the effectiveness of interventions offered. The Structured Assessment of Violence Risk in Youth (SAVRY) (Borum et al. 2002) assesses the risk of aggression based on a combination of historical and current factors, and also incorporates preservative or resilience factors as well as risk. It is designed to support structured professional judgement and has demonstrated good predictive validity in clinical practice (Meyers & Schmidt 2008; Dolan & Rennie, 2008). The Early Assessment Risk List for Boys (EARL-20B) (Augimeri et al. 2001) has been devised for violence risk assessment in younger boys, and there is also a version for girls called EARL-20G.

The Assessment, Intervention and Moving on (AIM) project is a structured assessment of the risk of sexually harmful behaviour developed in the UK (Print et al. 2007; Griffin et al. 2008). Other tools have been developed internationally, including the Estimate of Risk of Adolescent Sexual Offense Recidivism (ERASOR) (Worling 2004) and the

Juvenile Sex Offender Assessment Protocol-II (J-SOAP-II) (Prentky & Righthand 2003). These tools have some predictive validity, particularly when used in relation to the specific risk of sexual reoffending, rather than as general predictors of risk, but it is recommended that they are used as part of a broader strategy of risk assessment and management (Hempel et al. 2013). Such tools should only be used by specialised practitioners trained not only in the use of the tool but also in working with adolescents with sexually harmful behaviour. If the use of such a tool is being considered by a front line practitioner then consideration should be given to referring the young person to a more specialised service.

The most well known tools for assessing personality and its links with risk during adolescence are the Psychopathy Checklist: Youth Version (PCL: YV) (Forth et al. 2003), and the Millon Adolescent Clinical Inventory (MACI) (Millon, 1993). Other tools validated on adult populations have also been used for assessing older adolescents, such as the Structured Clinical Interview for DSM-IV Axis II Personality Disorders (SCID-II) (First et al. 1996). However, concerns have been raised regarding their developmental appropriateness (Seagrave & Grisso 2002), and the potential stigmatising effect of their use in clinical practice (Edens 2006).

There are some caveats and other factors that should be considered in relation to the use of risk assessment tools. First, although they may have some predictive validity in analysis of populations, there is also evidence that clinicians' risk judgements may have better predictors in clinical practice (Douglas et al. 2003; de Vogel et al. 2004). Second, adolescence is a time of major developmental change and judgements about risk should take this into consideration, particularly in relation to the use of personality measures (Dolan and Rennie 2008). Third, specialised tools for assessing particular areas of risk, such as sexual offending and fire setting, should only be used by trained practitioners working in specialised teams. Finally, robust risk assessment should also take resilience and preservative factors into consideration, as there is emerging evidence regarding their importance (Rennie & Dolan 2010).

Case management

Service user and carer involvement should be seen as central to the planning and delivery of care for young people in forensic settings, as in other CAMHS settings (Department of Health, 2004; Department of Health & Department for Children, Schools and Families, 2009). As well as being good practice, active engagement of service users is seen a key principle in achieving positive outcomes for young people with serious conduct problems (National Institution for Health and Clinical Excellence 2013).

All service provision and interventions for adolescent offenders need to be informed by robust case management practices, regardless of location. This is important, as in all CAMHS settings, in order to meet needs and ensure safe practice; however, in the forensic context it is also important from a public protection perspective. Case management in this context is more complex because the young people concerned have multiple needs, requiring multiple agency involvement and there is often an interplay between mental health needs and risk factors.

Case management must be informed by robust assessment processes that are regularly revisited and reviewed on a multidisciplinary basis. Decision making processes should be clear, transparent and well documented, and decisions about risk management should be based on good evidence to protect young people, the public and practitioners. Most importantly, case management in forensic CAMHS should incorporate information sharing processes with other agencies as a matter of routine. Information sharing practices between healthcare providers and other agencies (particularly those working in the justice field) have often been problematic in the past (Department of Health 2009), with healthcare professionals frequently citing medical confidentiality as a reason for not sharing information. Serious case reviews and inquiries repeatedly identify the failure to share information as a key factor in the breakdown of processes designed to protect children or the public (Ritchie et al. 1994; Department of Children Schools and Families 2010).

Actively engaging service users in the case management process is a key strategy for obtaining their consent to share information, but ultimately it is the duty of healthcare professionals to be aware of their responsibilities in this area and act accordingly; cross-agency guidance on information sharing has been drawn up by the Department of Health, Youth Justice Board, Ministry of Justice and the Department for Children, Schools and Families (Department of Health 2008).

Interventions

Mental health interventions for adolescent offenders should comply with the latest evidence and practice guidance relevant to the young person's identified needs. The treatment for mental health problems such as psychosis, depression or ADHD should be to the same standard as in any other setting, whether the intervention is psychological, pharmacological or social. The case management process should ensure that the additional factors of co-morbidity, case complexity and risk management can be addressed while still offering the young person high quality interventions.

However, most young people in contact with the justice system also present with significant conduct disorder, which is one of the factors complicating interventions for other mental health problems, and is also a problem that forensic CAMHS have a role in addressing. The strongest evidence base for interventions with preadolescent children is through the use of parenting programmes (Webster-Stratton 1984,1990), although there is some evidence for interventions directly with children themselves (Barkley et al. 2000). There have been more studies on interventions with preadolescent children, but the emerging evidence base suggests that the most effective interventions for conduct disorder in adolescence are via the immediate parent or carer system. For example, through therapeutic foster care (Baker et al. 2007; Hahn et al. 2005) or via wraparound multi-agency interventions such as multisystemic therapy (Henggeler et al. 1992, 1997).

Within the UK guidance on the assessment and management of conduct disorder is being drafted at the time of writing (National Institute for Health and Clinical Excellence 2013). However, the guidance for younger children is clear on recommending parenting interventions (National Institute for Health and Clinical Excellence 2006), although with the caveat that case complexity and the challenge of engaging young people and parents must be taken into consideration. The draft guidance outlines several key areas: improving pathways (including screening and comprehensive assessment), intervention early in the pathway, effective engagement of young people, families and agencies, robust case management processes (including coordinating care between agencies and sharing of information), and effective management of transitions.

If interventions for conduct disorder are viewed from a stepped care perspective then first stage interventions would be programmes addressing offending behaviour, decision making and social responsibility that are delivered via YOT workers and programme and intervention teams in secure settings. Interventions from mental health professionals would address associated mental health needs and contribute to the overall package to meet needs and manage risk. More severe conduct disorder may be directly associated with other mental health problems, meaning that mental health professionals would work to support the immediate care system (support and advice regarding care planning and the management of risk) as well as working directly with the young person. In the most serious cases, a comprehensive multi-agency approach is needed, whether in community or residential settings. If the offending or high-risk behaviours are particularly severe, such as sex offending, then mental health professionals should only be offering interventions for these (as opposed to other needs), as part of a specialised forensic service. In this model, forensic inpatient services would fulfil a similar function to other complex multi-agency interventions but focusing on young people whose profile of needs could not be met in other settings.

There is often a complex interplay between mental health needs and serious conduct disorder; in some cases the mental health needs are a direct contributor to offending behaviour (for instance a young person with psychosis who can be aggressive in response to auditory hallucinations). In many cases the link is indirect, but untreated mental health needs can be a risk factor for offending (for instance a young person who manages emotional dysregulation by substance misuse, which leads to aggression). In a small number of cases the mental health needs may mediate a strong underlying tendency to serious antisocial behaviour, and successful intervention for the mental health problem may lead to an increase in risk (for instance successful treatment for ADHD that increases the capacity for premeditation and planning to overcome obstacles to offending). A comprehensive approach to case management should help to anticipate how this interplay may work out and ensure that risk management strategies are effective.

Commissioning and delivering services

There have been significant changes over recent years in the context for service commissioning and delivery in the UK, and further change appears likely. In the community, the establishment of the Youth Justice Board in 1998 and the subsequent development of local YOTs created formal links for the first time between CAMHS and the justice system, thus enabling a pathway to mental health services for young offenders with mental health problems. In England medium secure inpatient services had been developed on an ad hoc basis but from 2002 were nationally commissioned to ensure adequate capacity and equity of access nationally. Prison mental health services came under the responsibility of local primary care trusts from 2005. Mental health provision into the rest of the young people's secure estate (i.e. within secure children's homes and secure training centres) will also come under the responsibility of local commissioners in the near future.

Community services

Although forensic CAMHS are commissioned within the general guidelines and principles that apply to all mental health services for young people, at the time of writing only medium secure inpatient services are being delivered to a standard specification and with agreed clinical standards. However, models for community forensic CAMHS and services in the secure estate are being developed. Therefore many current services tend to reflect local patterns of historical provision or to replicate models of service delivery from other areas, such as day services or outpatient clinics. So what would good forensic CAMHS provision look like in different settings?

Within community settings such as YOTs, mental health practitioners should be able to provide a first line of mental health assessment for young people as part of a comprehensive assessment of health needs that in turn links in to the young person's overall care and management. This part of the pathway should also include court liaison services and input into police custody suites. They should provide the link into local CAMHS for young people whose mental health needs require more specialist or multidisciplinary input, while at the same time remaining involved in order to facilitate the overall care and risk management of the young person, particularly for those young people with complex needs. The practitioner would identify and refer those young people whose profile of needs means that more specialist assessment and intervention may be necessary (for instance by a specialist forensic service). The role should also encompass support, consultation and training of the team regarding young people's mental health needs in general. To fulfil such a role, practitioners would require some training in risk assessment and management as well as a core skill set in adolescent mental health; they would not be expected to act as specialist practitioners but would require skills outside the normal range of CAMHS practitioners.

Secure settings

Within the secure estate, mental health provision should be configured to provide a comprehensive multidisciplinary service that would provide the following elements:

*   screening for common and potentially serious mental health problems as part of a comprehensive health screening process;
*   assessment, triage and liaison to identify those young people needing more specialist or multidisciplinary input;
*   robust case management and care planning processes that include information sharing with other agencies (including agencies involved in previous care, current care and any potential aftercare);
*   a range of more specialised multidisciplinary interventions including psychological, mental state monitoring, psycho-pharmacological and group interventions;

- joint working and consultation for young people with complex needs informed by the therapeutic parenting model;
- input into sentence planning and risk management for young people with complex needs and/or high-risk behaviours;
- a referral pathway to specialist forensic community teams and to medium secure inpatient services;
- support, training and consultation to other professionals and agencies within the establishment.

Case management, front line support for young people and carers, and information sharing are time-consuming but essential aspects of a comprehensive service, and can generally be delivered by experienced case workers such as nurses rather than by specialist practitioners, who should concentrate on the aspects of service delivery that no one else can deliver.

Adolescent boys, particularly those in contact with the justice system, are not renowned for their uptake of traditional mental health services, and models of service delivery in the secure estate should acknowledge this and adopt practices that have proven to be effective for other providers working with 'hard to reach' young people, typically third-sector providers. Services should adopt and adapt practices from assertive outreach to maximise accessibility and acceptability to prospective service users; a high profile approach is needed that embeds mental health provision into the daily structures and routines of the establishment, rather than being a stand-alone service. Such an approach demystifies mental health and directly increases the accessibility (and therefore approachability) of front line mental health practitioners.

Highly specialised community and inpatient forensic CAMHS

Dedicated community and inpatient forensic CAMHS play a key role in the pathway for young people with serious mental health problems and high-risk behaviours; they need robust links with the other agencies earlier in the pathway if they are to provide consultations, assessments and interventions in an accessible and timely manner. They should comprise multidisciplinary teams with highly specialist knowledge and expertise unlikely to be available within other services working with this population. Specialist forensic CAMHS are likely to serve large populations and may cover large geographical areas. Maintaining effective pathways and links with multiple partner agencies under these circumstances is a challenge, and links with key agencies such as YOT teams, CAMHS and secure establishments is a priority.

Community forensic CAMHS should be configured to deliver services in line with the recently developed draft service specification, which may provide the template for future commissioning. These roles should include:

- highly specialist forensic mental health triage, including advice and signposting and formal consultation;
- support for local services in high-risk cases through multi-agency care-planning;

- reduction and management of risk through comprehensive risk assessment and individualised treatment plans;
- specialist forensic mental health assessment and intervention in high-risk cases;
- where appropriate, ensure evidence-based treatment for complex high-risk cases, through a wide range of interventions, to address individual's mental health, welfare and educational needs;
- coordination of, and liaison with, mental health services across community and custodial settings;
- development of joint working arrangements with partner agencies, including specialist training packages and transition arrangements with services for young people and adults;
- informing and developing strategic links between mental health services and the youth justice system at the regional and national levels.

Inpatient services already have an established service specification and clinical standards. The services have to meet standards in three key areas:

1   As adolescent services they have to provide developmentally appropriate care attuned to the complex needs their service users typically present with; it needs to facilitate the young person's emotional, cognitive, moral, educational and social development.
2   As forensic services they have to provide a secure and safe environment that can effectively manage high-risk and often high-cost behaviours and at the same time manage high levels of vulnerability.
3   As mental health services they have to provide comprehensive multifaceted evidence-based treatments and evaluate their effectiveness.

High quality service delivery is essential in all three areas; to compromise the quality of care in order to maintain security (for instance) would not be acceptable. As highly specialised services, both community and inpatient forensic CAMHS are expected to be at the forefront of innovation and service development. Consequently they should have a key role in research and inform future models of service delivery and policy development.

Workforce and training issues

Forensic CAMHS has developed significantly over recent years and is continuing to evolve. The original scope of the term was taken to include only highly specialised inpatient and community services operating at Tier 4. However, it has become increasingly clear that practitioners at all tiers within the system have training needs arising from the complex nature of the field. It has been proposed that forensic CAMHS represents a combination of concepts and models from two different fields: forensic mental health and child and adolescent mental health. For many practitioners their pathway into forensic CAMHS is via one of these two routes, but rarely via both. Thus many practitioners in the field begin with a knowledge base and skill set that does not encompass all the relevant domains.

For many practitioners the solution to this problem is to seek out and undertake training in the areas currently missing from their knowledge and skill framework. This may take the form of specific training to explicitly address an area such as the use of a risk assessment tool, or more comprehensive training, probably at post-graduate level, to acquire a more thorough grounding in child and adolescent mental health or forensic mental health. While this strategy is helpful to individual practitioners, at least three problems arise. First, it relies on individual practitioners to identify and meet their own training needs, which will be achieved in a non-standard way. Second, if forensic CAMHS represents a synthesis of concepts from the two separate fields, then this should be represented in the training, i.e. both forensic and CAMHS concepts and practice in one package. Third, this ad hoc approach will fail to address the longer-term needs of building workforce capacity in this area – only a more systematic approach will achieve this. To be accessible nationally, such training would need to be available at multiple sites and utilise distance learning as much as possible. Thematically the training should include, amongst other things:

- child development and attachment (including trauma);
- adolescent mental health needs and interventions, including psychosis, emotional disorders, ADHD, neuro-developmental disorders, conduct disorder, personality disorder;
- therapeutic parenting;
- risk assessment and management;
- personality development and pathways through services.

Such a list is not exclusive but is a starting point for a training programme geared towards future workforce development.

Conclusion

Services for young people in forensic settings are still at an early stage of development and further change into the future is inevitable; this constitutes an opportunity for further innovation in interventions and models of service delivery. Commissioners, service directors and clinicians will have to be creative in their approach, adapting models from other settings when appropriate but also being prepared to commit resources to innovative projects in order to meet the needs of this population.

References

Abram, KM, Teplin, LA, McClelland, GM & Dulcan, MK (2003) Comorbid psychiatric disorders in youth in juvenile detention. *Archives of General Psychiatry*, 60, 1097–1108.

Augimeri, L, Webster, C, Koegl, C & Levene, K (2001) *Early Assessment Risk List for Boys: EARL-20B*, Version 2. Toronto: Earlscourt Child and Family Centre.

Bailey, S, Doreleijers, T & Tarbuck, P (2006) Recent developments in mental health screening and assessment in juvenile justice systems. *Child and Adolescent Psychiatric Clinics of North America*, 15(2), 391–406.

Bailey, S, Pederson, C, Losel, F & Vermieren, R (2007) *Second Expert Paper: Antisocial personality disorder: children and adolescents mental illness and serious harm to others*. NHS National Programme on Forensic Mental Health Research and Development. Retrieved 20 May 2011, from www.liv. ac.uk/fmhweb/EP%20Anti%20social%20Personality%20Disorder%20Children.pdf

Bailey, S, Shaw, J, Tarbuck, P, Verstrecken, P, Turner, O, Law, H & Tonak, D (2008) *Mental Health Care Pathways for Juveniles and Young Persons in the Criminal Justice System*. London: Department of Health, unpublished.

Baker, AJ, Kurland, D, Curtis, P, Alexander, G. & Papa-Lentini, C (2007) Mental health and behavioral problems of youth in the child welfare system: residential treatment centers compared to therapeutic foster care in the Odyssey Project population. *Child Welfare*, 86(3), 97–123.

Barkley, RA, Shelton, TL, Crosswait, C, Moorehouse, M, Fletcher, K, Barrett, S, Jenkins, L. & Metevia, L (2000) Multi-method psycho-educational intervention for preschool children with disruptive behavior: preliminary results at post-treatment. *Journal of Child Psychology and Psychiatry and Allied Disciplines*, 41, 319–332.

Borum, R, Bartel, P & Forth, A (2002) *Manual for the Structured Assessment of Violence Risk in Youth (SAVRY)*. Tampa, FL: Florida Mental Health Institute.

Briere, J (1996) *Trauma Symptom Checklist for Children: Professional manual*. Odessa: Psychological Assessment Resources, Inc.

Bryan, K, Freer, J, & Furlong, C (2007) Language and communication difficulties in juvenile offenders. *International Journal of Language and Communication Disorders*, 42, 505–520.

Chitsabesan, P, Kroll, L, Bailey, S, Kenning, C, Sneider, S, MacDonald, W & Theodosiou, L (2006) Mental health needs of young offenders in custody and in the community. *British Journal of Psychiatry*, 188, 534–540.

Chitsabesan, P, Rothwell, J, Kenning, C, Law, H, Carter, L-A, Bailey, S & Clarke, A (2012) Six years on: a prospective cohort study of male juvenile offenders in secure care. *European Child and Adolescent Psychiatry*, 21(6), 339–347.

Conners, CK, Sitarenios, G, Parker, JDA. & Epstein, JN (1998) The Revised Conners' Parent Rating Scale (CPRS-R): factor structure, reliability, and criterion validity. *Journal of Abnormal Child Psychology*, 26(4), 257–268.

Costello, EJ, Angold, A, Burns, BJ, Stangl, DK, Tweed, DL, Erkanli, A & Worthman, CM (1996) The Great Smoky Mountains Study of youth – goals, design, methods, and the prevalence of DSM-III-R disorders. *Archives of General Psychiatry*, 53, 1129–1136.

de Vogel, V, de Ruiter, C, van Beek, D, & Mead, G (2004) Predictive validity of the SVR-20 and Static-99 in a Dutch sample of treated sex offenders. *Law and Human Behavior*, 28, 235–251.

Department for Children, Schools and Families (2010) *Working Together to Safeguard Children: A guide to inter-agency working to safeguard and promote the welfare of children*. Nottingham: DCSF Publications.

Department for Children, Schools and Families & Department of Health (2009) *CAMHS Review: Children and young people in mind*. London: Crown Publications.

Department of Health (2004) *The National Service Framework for Children, Young People and Maternity Services: The mental health and emotional well-being of children and young people*. London: Department of Health.

Department of Health (2008) *When to Share Information: Best practice guidance for everyone working in the youth justice system*. London: Department of Health.

Department of Health. (2009) *The Bradley Report: Lord Bradley's review of people with mental health problems or learning disabilities in the criminal justice system*. London: Department of Health Publications.

Department of Health & Department for Children, Schools and Families (2009) *Improving Access to Child and Adolescent Mental Health Services*. London: Department of Health Publications.

Dolan, M, & Rennie, C (2008) The Structured Assessment of Violence Risk in Youth (SAVRY) as a predictor of recidivism in a UK cohort of adolescent offenders with conduct disorder. *Psychological Assessment*, 20, 35–46.

Doreleijers, TAH, Boonmann, C, van Loosbroek, E, & Vermeiren, RRJM (2011) Assessing the psychometric properties and the perceived usefulness of the BasisRaadsOnderzoek (BARO) as a first-line screening instrument for juvenile offenders. *Child and Adolescent Psychiatry and Mental Health*, 5, 24, 1–7.

Douglas, KS, Ogloff, JRP & Hart, SD (2003) Evaluation of a model of risk assessment among forensic psychiatric patients. *Psychiatric Services*, 54, 1372–1379.

Edens, JF (2006) Unresolved controversies concerning psychopathy: implications for clinical and forensic decision-making. *Professional Psychology: Research and Practice*, 37, 59–65.

First, MB, Spitzer, RL, Gibbon, M & Williams, J (1996) *Structured Clinical Interview for DSM-IV (SCID-II)*. New York: Biometrics Research Department, New York State Psychiatric Institute.

Forth, AE, Kosson, DS & Hare, RD (2003) *The Psychopathy Checklist: Youth version manual*. Toronto: Multi-Health Systems.

Gasquet, I, Chavance, M, Ledoux, S & Choquet, M (1997) Psychosocial factors associated with help-seeking behavior among depressive adolescents. *European Child and Adolescent Psychiatry*, 6, 151–159.

Griffin, HL, Beech, A, Print, B, Bradshaw, H & Quayle, J (2008) The development and initial testing of the AIM2 framework to assess risk and strengths in young people who sexually offend. *Journal of Sexual Aggression*, 14, 211–225.

Grisso, T, Barnum, R, Fletcher, KE, Cauffman, E & Peuschold, D (2001) Massachusetts Youth Screening Instrument for mental health needs of juvenile justice youths. *Journal of the American Academy of Child and Adolescent Psychiatry*, 40(5), 541–548.

Hahn, RA, Bilukha, O, Lowy, J, Crosby, A, Fullilove, MT, Liberman, A, Moscicki, E, Snyder, S, Tuma, F, Corso, P & Schofield, A (2005) The effectiveness of therapeutic foster care for the prevention of violence: a systematic review. *American Journal of Preventive Medicine*, 28, 72– 90.

Hall, I (2000) Young offenders with a learning disability. *Advances in Psychiatric Treatment*, 6, 278–285.

Hempel, I, Buck, N, Cima, M & van Marle, H (2013) Review of risk assessment instruments for juvenile sex offenders. *International Journal of Offender Therapy and Comparative Criminology*, 57(2), 208–228.

Henggeler, SW, Melton, GB & Smith, LA (1992) Family preservation using multisystemic therapy: an effective alternative to incarcerating serious juvenile offenders. *Journal of Consulting and Clinical Psychology*, 60, 953–961.

Henggeler, SW, Melton, GB, Brondino, MJ, Sherer, DG & Hanley, JH (1997) Multisystemic therapy with violent and chronic juvenile offenders and their families: the role of treatment fidelity in successful dissemination. *Journal of Consulting and Clinical Psychology*, 65, 821–833.

HM Prison Service & NHS Executive (1999) *The Future Organisation of Prison Health Care*. Report by the Joint Prison Service and National Health Service Executive Working Group. London: Department of Health.

Hoare, T & Wilson, J (2010) *Directory of Services for High-risk Young People*. London: Centre for Mental Health.

Ireland, JL, Boustead, R & Ireland, CA (2005) Coping style and psychological health among adolescent prisoners: a study of young and juvenile offenders. *Journal of Adolescence*, 28, 411–423.

Kaufman, J, Birmaher, B, Brent, D, Rao, U, Flynn, C, Moreci, P, Williamson, D & Ryan, N (1997) Schedule for affective disorders and schizophrenia for school-age children present and lifetime version (K-SADS-PL): initial reliability and validity data. *Journal of the American Academy of Child and Adolescent Psychiatry*, 36(7), 980–988.

Khan, L (2010) *Reaching Out, Reaching In: Promoting mental health and emotional well-being in secure settings*. London: Centre for Mental Health.

Krawiecka, M, Goldberg, D & Vaughan, M (1977) Standardised psychiatric assessment scale for chronic psychotic patients. *Acta Psychiatrica Scandinavia*, 36, 25–31.

Kroll, L, Woodham, A, Rothwell, J, Bailey, S, Tobias, C, Harrington, R & Marshall, M (1999) Reliability of the Salford needs assessment schedule for adolescents. *Psychological Medicine*, 29, 891–902.

Kroll, L, Rothwell, J, Bradley, D, Shah, P, Bailey, S & Harrington, R (2002) Mental health needs of *boys in secure care for serious or persistent offending: a prospective longitudinal study. The Lancet*, 359, 1975–1979.

Lader, D, Singleton, N & Meltzer, H (2000) *Psychiatric Morbidity among Young Offenders in England and Wales. Further analysis of data from the ONS survey*. London: Home Office.

MacReady, N (2009) US faces crisis in mental health care for juvenile offenders. *The Lancet*, 374, 601.

Maughan, B & Kim-Cohen, J (2005) Continuities between childhood and adult life. *British Journal of Psychiatry*, 187, 605–617.

Meltzer, H, Gatward, H, Goodman, R & Ford, T (2000) *Mental Health of Children and Adolescents in Great Britain*. London: The Stationery Office.

Meyers, JR & Schmidt, F (2008) Predictive Validity of the Structured Assessment for Violence Risk in Youth (SAVRY) with juvenile offenders. *Criminal Justice and Behavior*. 35(3), 344–355.

Millon, T (1993) *Millon Adolescent Clinical Inventory Manual*. Minneapolis, MN: National Computer Systems.

Mitchell, P (2006) Adolescent forensic mental health nursing. In: McDougall, T (ed.). *Child and Adolescent Mental Health Nursing*. London: Blackwell.

Mitchell, P & Shaw, J (2011) Factors affecting the recognition of mental health problems amongst adolescent offenders in custody. *Journal of Forensic Psychiatry and Psychology*, 22(3), 381–394.

National Institute for Health and Clinical Excellence & Social Care Institute for Excellence (2006) *Nice Technology Appraisal 102: Parent-training/education programmes in the management of children with conduct disorders*. London: National Institute for Health and Clinical Excellence.

National Institute for Health and Clinical Excellence (2009) *Antisocial Personality Disorder; the NICE guideline on treatment, management and prevention*. London: National Institute for Health and Clinical Excellence.

National Institute for Health and Clinical Excellence (2013) *Conduct Disorders and Antisocial Behaviour in Children and Young People: recognition, intervention and management*. London: National Institute for Health and Clinical Excellence.

Office of the Children's Commissioner (2011) *I Think I Must Have Been Born Bad: Emotional health and wellbeing of children and young people in the youth justice system*. London: Office of the Children's Commissioner.

Parke, S (2009) *Children and Young People in Custody 2006–2008: An analysis of the experiences of 15–18-year-olds in prison*. London: HM Inspector of Prisons/Youth Justice Board.

Prentky, R & Righthand, S (2003) Juvenile Sex Offender Assessment Protocol-II (J-SOAP-II). Retrieved February 2013, from http://www.psicologiagiuridica.eu/files/didattica/jsoap2.pdf

Print, B, Griffin, H, Beech, AR, Quayle, J, Bradshaw, H, Henniker, J & Morrison, T (2007) *AIM2: An initial assessment model for young people who display sexually harmful behaviour*. Manchester: AIM Project.

Rennie, C & Dolan, M (2010) The significance of protective factors in the assessment of risk. *Criminal Behaviour and Mental Health*, 20, 8–22.

Ritchie, JH, Dick, D & Lingham, R (1994) *The Report of the Inquiry into the Care and Treatment of Christopher Clunis*. London: HMSO.

Rutter, M, Giller, H & Hagell, A (1998) *Antisocial Behaviour by Young People*. Cambridge: Cambridge University Press.

Ryan, T & Mitchell, P (2011) A collaborative approach to meeting the needs of adolescent offenders with complex needs in custodial settings: an 18 month cohort study. *Journal of Forensic Psychiatry and Psychology*, 22(3), 437–454.

Sayal, K, Taylor, E, Beecham, J & Byrne, P (2002) Pathways to care in children at risk of attention-deficit hyperactivity disorder. *British Journal of Psychiatry*, 18, 43–48.

Seagrave, D & Grisso, T (2002) Adolescent development and the measurement of juvenile psychopathy. *Law and Human Behavior*, 26, 219–239.

Shelton, D (2004) Experiences of detained young offenders in need of mental health care. *Journal of Nursing Scholarship*, 36(2), 129–133.

Teplin, LA, Abram, KM, McClelland, GM, Dulcan, MK & Mericle, AA (2002) Psychiatric disorders in youth in juvenile detention. *Archives of General Psychiatry*, 59, 1133–1143.

Vermeiren, R, Jespers, I & Moffitt, TE (2006) Mental health problems in juvenile justice populations. *Child and Adolescent Psychiatric Clinics of North America*, 15, 333–352.

Vreugdenhil, C, Doreleijers, TAH, Vermeiren, R, Wouters, LFJM & van den Brink, W (2004) Psychiatric disorders in a representative sample of incarcerated boys in the Netherlands. *Journal of the American Academy of Child and Adolescent Psychiatry*, 43, 97–104.

Webster-Stratton, C (1984) Randomized trial of two parent-training programs for families with conduct-disordered children. *Journal of Consulting and Clinical Psychology*, 52, 666–678.

Webster-Stratton, C (1990) Long-term follow-up of families with young conduct problem children: from preschool to grade school. *Journal of Clinical Child Psychology*, 19, 144–149.

Whittle, N, Macdonald, W & Bailey, S (in press). 'I'm just the boy in number twenty to the officers': a study of young offenders' perceptions of health and healthcare services in custody and in the community. *International Journal of Correctional Healthcare*.

Williams, R & Kerfoot, M (2005) *Child and Adolescent Mental Health Services: Strategy, planning, delivery, and evaluation*. Oxford: Oxford University Press.

Withecomb, J (2008) Adolescent forensic psychiatry. *Psychiatry*, 7(9), 395–398.

Withecomb, J & Jasti, MP (2007) Adolescent forensic psychiatry. *Psychiatry*, 6(10), 424–428.

Worling, JR (2004) The Estimate of Risk of Adolescent Sexual Offense Recidivism (ERASOR): preliminary psychometric data. *Sexual Abuse: A Journal of Research and Treatment*, 16(3), 235–254.

Youth Justice Board (2007) *Accommodation Needs and Experiences: A summary of research commissioned by the Youth Justice Board for England and Wales (YJB) into the housing needs and experiences of young people who have offended*. London: Youth Justice Board.

Youth Justice Board (2012) *Youth Justice Statistics 2010-11*. London, Youth Justice Board.

Zimmer-Gembeck, MJ & Locke, EM (2007) The socialization of adolescent coping behaviours: relationships with family and teachers. *Journal of Adolescence*, 30, 1–16.

Zwaanswijk, M, Van der Ende, J, Verhaak, PFM, Bensing, JM & Verhulst, FC (2003) Factors associated with adolescent mental health service need and utilization. *Journal of the American Academy of Child and Adolescent Psychiatry*, 42, 692–700.

10

CHILDREN AND YOUNG PEOPLE'S VIEWS OF SERVICES

What they say and why it matters

Cathy Street

Key points

- The views of children and young people must be sought and taken in to account when planning, improving and evaluating services.
- The available research on participation and involvement shows that young people, their parents and healthcare providers often have different views and expectations of services.
- Young people want access to better information about services. This should be offered in a variety of formats and helps enable greater involvement in care and treatment decisions.
- Young people want help from professionals who are non-judgemental, empathetic, respectful, open-minded, informed, competent and respecting of their privacy and confidentiality.
- Young people in hospital want access to a range of individual and group-based activities alongside support with their education. They also want help with the development of skills to help them leave hospital and get on with their lives.

Introduction

For such an important part of Child and Adolescent Mental Health Services (CAMHS), the literature concerning the views of the children, young people, and families and carers who use Tier 4 services is quite limited (National Institute for Health Research 2008). In part, this may reflect the small numbers of children and young people requiring the most specialist CAMHS; however, many of the research studies and service evaluations that have presented children and young people's views relate to CAMHS in general and have not attempted to make any 'cross tier' comparisons or to be 'tier specific'.

Overview

In general, existing literature has looked at young people's views of staff working in health services more broadly. Some studies have explored the barriers children and young people can face in accessing mental healthcare, with young people's experiences during the transition from CAMHS to other services, notably adult mental health services (AMHS) attracting increasing attention in recent years. A few studies have sought children and young people's views about what are sometimes termed 'alternatives to Tier 4' and some have addressed young people's experiences of inappropriate admissions to adult inpatient care. The issue of children and young people's involvement and participation in mental healthcare also provides some valuable information about mental health service provision from the perspective of children and young people, and makes the case for why it is important to seek the views of, and listen to, those using CAMHS at whatever tier.

The only sizeable study identified specific to Tier 4 CAMHS and with a specific focus on giving young people 'a voice' identified is the YoungMinds study *Where Next? New directions in inpatient mental health services for young people* (Dogra 2005; Street 2004) which gathered information from 107 young people and 35 parents, and a much smaller study of intensive home treatment (Farnfield & Kaznap 1998) where 7 young people and 12 parents shared their views about the service.

In order to address this paucity of information, this chapter therefore draws upon a number of different and sometimes not formally published sources. These include some unpublished feedback from children and young people provided to the National Youth Advocacy Service (NYAS) who offer annual inspection visits to a number of inpatient CAMHS units in England; feedback gathered by inpatient staff undertaking their own in-house service evaluations; and selected data relating to Tier 4 services from CHASE, the Child and Adolescent Service Experience psychometric tool which is now in routine use across a British mental health trust. CHASE was developed to improve children and young people's experience of mental healthcare and the participation of young people was built into its development throughout to ensure that the tool reflects their priorities as distinct from the views of their parents or mental health practitioners.

Mental health services – what children and young people have said

Nisha Dogra's (2005) review of the literature concerning children and young people's views on CAMHS begins by highlighting the limited amount of literature and also noting weaknesses in some of the studies undertaken. He also reports limited evidence of young people's involvement in healthcare actually happening in practice. Dogra's conclusion is that, despite its limitations, the available research shows that young people, their parents and healthcare providers often have different expectations of services. Young people want accessible services staffed by those they are able to trust and who demonstrate an ability to listen. Above all, young people want to be involved in the decisions about them (Dogra 2005).

Many of the themes discussed in Dogra's review echo those described in a National Children's Bureau 'highlight' on this topic (Street 2004). This summarises some of the earlier literature from the late 1990s and early 2000s including work by Farnfield & Kaznap

(1998), Buston (2002), Gibson & Possamai (2002) and Boylan (2004). These studies emphasised the importance of young people feeling that their views were being listened to, and of having staff in mental health services who are available, approachable, empathetic and able to make things happen. Possession of such skills was also found to be more important than the actual profession of the staff member.

Children and young people's views of health professionals are also explored in a study by Sherman-Jones (2003) who looked at young people's perception of and access to health advice, and the review of 31 research studies published between 2000 and 2009 undertaken by Robinson (2010). Sherman-Jones' work raised issues about the need for confidential, accessible and non-judgemental health advice and services delivered from accessible settings. In the review by Robinson, it is reported that the themes emerging from the children and young people's views comprised wanting health professionals to be familiar, accessible and available; to be informed and competent; to provide accessible information; to be a good communicator; to participate in care; to ensure privacy and confidentiality; and to demonstrate acceptance and empathy. Robinson makes the point that the wish expressed by children and young people to have informed and competent health professionals, who understood their illness, sometimes arose out of their negative experiences. In her conclusion, Robinson notes that her findings are strikingly similar to other studies of children and young people's views of professionals, including of the workforce in general (Department for Children, Schools and Families 2008) and of what is a 'good nurse' (Brady 2009).

Findings from the National Advisory Council for Children's Mental Health and Psychological Wellbeing Young People's Reference Group

The National Advisory Council (NAC) for Children's Mental Health and Psychological Wellbeing came into being as a direct result of a national review of CAMHS (Department for Children, Schools and Families & Department of Health 2008). It was created as a new national body to hold the government to account for delivering the CAMHS review recommendations and to champion children and young people's emotional well-being and mental health. A Young People's Reference Group informed its work, and the group's views of CAMHS were published in 2011 in a briefing paper with the frustrated title of *How Many Times Do We Have to Tell You?* (Lavis & Hewson 2011).

Based partly on a short literature review which looked at papers and reports published within the last 10 years involving consultations with children and young people, and backed by a series of meetings with the Reference Group, the briefing paper's overview of what young people think about mental health services identified the following:

- Young people want holistic services, based in convenient locations, which meet their mental health needs but which also provide access to a range of other help and support.
- Services need to be accessible and flexible, with the opportunity to take part in activities that are fun and creative and which can help them build a range of softer skills such as building friendships.

- Long wait times are a deterrent to young people who want quicker access to help in an emergency, better out-of-hours and crisis support and more accessible inpatient provision.
- The importance of services being friendly, welcoming, offering a safe, clean and homely environment; wherein the attitude of staff was seen to be crucial.
- TServices need to be age-appropriate.

The NAC briefing paper reviews the barriers young people identified to accessing mental health services. In particular, the stigma associated with mental health, concerns about confidentiality, previous bad experiences of services and a lack of information about services were highlighted as important. The briefing also highlights the importance young people attach to choice and informed consent, and to the provision of information and communication between services. In particular, the need for better communication between inpatient units and community CAMHS was emphasised by a number of the Reference Group members.

Other prominent themes concerned young people's participation, and the importance of the relationship between young people and the staff caring for them. Notably, the need for trust to be established in this relationship and of improving transitional planning and care were strong messages. The paper also describes the findings of a large scale consultation event with children and young people which looked at the attributes they identified as making the 'perfect worker'. In keeping with a number of other studies, the attributes identified included staff being non-judgemental, empathetic, respectful, open-minded, informed, competent and alert to ensuring that privacy and confidentiality are respected.

Children and young people's involvement in CAMHS – why seeking their views is important

A number of studies have explored children and young people's participation in mental health services, or have examined the barriers that impede children and young people sharing their views about services (Day 2008; Worrall-Davies 2008). Interest in this area reflects the increasing prominence in health policy and guidance given to the views of service users having a key role in driving forward service improvement. For children and young people this involves helping to develop better child or young person-centred care and treatment interventions and services.

In her study of the barriers and facilitators to children's and young people's views affecting the planning and delivery of CAMHS, Worrall-Davies (2008) cites the work of Sinclair (2004). This identifies three main factors as the drivers behind the importance given to children and young people's involvement in services. These are the growing influence of the consumer in society; the children's rights agenda; and new social science research that promotes better understanding of children and young people as agents rather than passive recipients of social change (Sinclair 2004).

In her review of best practice in seeking the views of children and young people, Worrall-Davies argues that it is crucial that we understand from children and young people how they feel about receiving care and treatment from CAMHS (Worrall-Davies 2008). She also cites

Main (2006) who, in a paper entitled 'The Future of Mental Health', predicted that the future balance of power will no longer be so much within the system, but instead be based more on equal partnership between services and the individual who uses, or even chooses, them.

Day's exploration of children's and young people's involvement and participation in mental healthcare aims to highlight children and young people's unique contribution to clinical care and examine current knowledge and practice that encourages their involvement in clinical processes and service development (Day 2008). Day highlights that the National Service Framework (NSF) for Children, Young People and Maternity Services (Department of Health 2004) emphasises that the views of children (including very young children), young people, parents and carers must be sought and taken in to account when planning, improving and evaluating services. Day also draws attention to the need for a proactive approach to ensure the involvement of socially excluded groups. Indeed, one of the NSF 'markers of good practice' is practitioners having the requisite skills to communicate directly with children and young people.

In his examination of the aims and objectives of children and young people's participation, Day (2008) also highlights the value of service user views in improving the quality and effectiveness of services. These, he suggests, can be used to improve service uptake and engagement, clinical knowledge and decision making as well as shape interventions and provision so that they better reflect children and young people's own concerns and priorities. Additionally, in the section of the paper focusing on children and young people's unique contributions, Day makes a number of points which illustrate why listening to children and young people about their experiences of mental health services matters. He highlights what may sometime emerge as 'discrepancies' between the child or young person and their parents or carers, as well as differences in perspectives between professionals and families on the nature of the mental health difficulties, the reasons for referral and the treatment or therapy goals. Day reinforces the message that service users feel more involved in their care when they are treated as equal partners, listened to and properly informed (Day 2008).

Paul (2004) examines the ethics of children and young people making decisions about their mental healthcare. The findings suggest that children and young people should receive accurate information in appropriate formats, be encouraged to express their views and to contribute to discussions about their needs. They also need to be able to take an informed role in making decisions about their treatment and care, including the best available interventions, their likely benefits, risks and possible alternatives. Young people should also have access to developmentally appropriate, personally relevant, accurate information in usable forms to assist involvement in their own mental healthcare (Day 2008).

Lessons from research exploring mental health service transitions

A central theme of the National CAMHS Review (Department for Children, Schools and Families & Department of Health 2008) and the related work of the National Advisory Council has been the need to improve transitional care for young people, in particular for those aged 16–18 requiring a move to adult mental health services. Whilst not specifically focused on Tier 4 provision, some of the research in this area has explored young people's experiences and views of the inpatient services they received and provides valuable insights into what young people in transition find helpful, or want from mental health services.

One study that sought to better understand young people's experiences of transition is the work of Munoz-Solomando and colleagues. This review highlights the importance of services working in a way that includes active steps to promote a young person's autonomy. This is based on the premise that young people who have mental health disorders may experience more problems in achieving autonomy than their contemporaries. Munoz-Solomando's review also reiterates the need for service developments to be based on the needs of the young people who use them rather than the professionals that provide them. This is crucially important when we consider that perceptions of need held by young people and parents about the services offered to them are sometimes very different from those of practitioners. A key recommendation from this work is that mental health services need to be responsive to the varying and diverse range of needs typically presented by young people in the transition age range (Munoz-Solomando et al. 2010). This principle has also been applied to mental health services for young people in the US where researchers have suggested that a gradual transition is critical for the experience to be as positive as possible for young people at such an unpredictable and vulnerable time in their lives (Manteuffel et al. 2008).

The Transition from CAMHS to Adult Mental Health Services (TRACK) study explored the experiences of seventy-nine young people from across six areas of London and the West Midlands (Singh et al. 2009). Drawing out the qualitative experiences of young people in the TRACK study, Hovish et al. (2012) highlighted the multiple health and social care needs typically presented by young people in transition between mental health services, and cited multi-agency service involvement as the norm. The issue of transition in hospital, community and home-based services is explored further in the following chapter.

Young people on adult mental health wards

One area of mental health service provision for children and young people which has attracted a lot of political and media attention has been inappropriate admission to adult mental health wards (McDougall & Bodley-Scott 2008). In 2007, a report by the Office of the Children's Commissioner for England called *Pushed into the Shadows* drew attention to the poor levels of care often experienced by young people admitted to adult inpatient mental health facilities (Office of the Children's Commissioner 2007). Since that time, the law has changed, with accompanying government guidance making it clear that children and young people should be only be admitted to age appropriate settings (National Institute for Mental Health in England 2009). Nevertheless, some of the views expressed by young people in *Pushed into the Shadows* are clearly pertinent to understanding young people's experiences and views about inpatient mental healthcare.

The research for the report that went to the Children's Commissioner for England was undertaken by a small team of consultants and researchers from YoungMinds. They explored the journeys of 16 young people between the ages of 13 and 19 who had required inpatient mental healthcare and who, for a variety of reasons, had been placed on an adult ward. Most of the young people were interviewed after discharge, although one was still an inpatient and two were in specialist residential therapeutic placements that had been organised for them on discharge from an adult ward. The young people consulted for this work made a number of specific recommendations including the need for mental health units and staff to be able to:

*   respond more quickly;
*   address the wide range of needs young people typically have;
*   offer a high level of security with staff who have expertise in managing challenging behaviour.

Young people also highlighted the importance of age-appropriate provision. They told researchers that being in a unit with people their own age was really important and that having opportunities to do things with young people experiencing similar difficulties was essential. The provision of information and supporting young people to be fully involved in their care and discharge planning were other prominent themes. *Pushed into the Shadows* noted that independent advice and advocacy support was something all young people who are admitted to mental health inpatient facilities should have access to. In terms of daily routines, the young people were quite clear that inpatient care needed to include a programme of regular daily activities and to provide education. Several of the group had experienced admissions to both CAMHS and adult wards, and pointed out the differences to researchers. On the whole, young people felt that CAMHS units had a more relaxed atmosphere with more activities and groups, and it was easier for their family and friends to visit.

What young people say specifically about Tier 4 CAMHS

YoungMinds *Where Next?* study (Street & Svanberg 2003) explored young people's views and experiences of inpatient care, with the main sample being drawn from young people who were resident in six CAMHS units. The study was supplemented by some information from young people who had been admitted to paediatric wards and some retrospective data which was collected by postal questionnaire from young people who had been discharged in the six-month period prior to the study commencing.

The average age of the respondents in the *Where Next?* study was 16.4 years and they had a range of diagnoses including psychosis, depression, eating disorder, post-traumatic stress disorder (PTSD) and personality disorder. The study findings touched on many different areas of inpatient care, right from the stage of an admission being offered through to discharge. A prominent theme running throughout all the comments noted by young people was about access to information. This, young people said, should be offered in a variety of formats, including both verbal explanations and written material. Young people were also clear in stating their wish to be involved in the decision making about their care.

With regard to how admission was managed, within the *Where Next* sample, 8 per cent had positive views about admission. However, 26 per cent reported a negative experience, with 25 per cent feeling isolated or unsupported, 20 per cent feeling frightened, 10 per cent feeling trapped and 10 per cent missing home. A fifth of the sample mentioned the distance they had been placed from home, of which 69 per cent found too far away.

The prominent issues and concerns raised by young people in the *Where Next?* study are to a large extent similar to the studies mentioned earlier about CAMHS in general, namely:

- the importance of care that is age-appropriate, flexible and responsive to young people's individual needs;
- of having staff who are available, approachable, empathetic and skilled in listening to young people;
- of units being non-institutional, 'homely', clean, well-decorated and fully equipped;
- of inpatient programmes offering daily activities, including education and both individual and group-based activities (especially since boredom was highlighted by a number of those interviewed).

The need for privacy and personal space, for clarity around consent and confidentiality of information, and for young units providing a safe environment, were also regularly raised in the study interviews and focus groups. Other positive aspects of Tier 4 services identified by young people included:

- access to staff who were properly trained to support young people with complex needs;
- group-based activities and opportunities to do things with other young people;
- supported education and help with the development of coping skills and moving on;
- support at night.

However, these aspects of inpatient care were not universally viewed as positive. For example, some young people reported unhelpful group dynamics and experiences of peer pressure. Some had not experienced any consistency in the support offered by unit staff, and others reported a high staff turnover and use of agency and bank nursing staff. Several felt that the education provision was inadequate, with poor liaison with their own school, and a fairly widespread complaint was of inadequate and poorly coordinated discharge planning.

Box 10.1 includes some key messages from the *Where Next?* study, highlighting the views of young people about Tier 4 inpatient services.

Young people's views about intensive community and home treatment services

A study by Rani and colleagues (2009) explored user and carer views of intensive home treatment. This reflects the growing interest in what are sometimes called 'alternatives' to Tier 4 inpatient provision. In explaining that there is growing evidence that some intensive community treatments, notably assertive outreach, can be as effective as inpatient mental healthcare for some young people, Rani et al. note that there is very little known about the experiences of young people and families in receipt of these services.

To address this gap in knowledge, Rani and colleagues therefore decided to interview a sample of young service users of an intensive home treatment service, and their parents, in order to obtain a descriptive account of their views and experiences of the service within the context of the framework of innovative and alternative models of CAMHS Tier 4

BOX 10.1   What young people said about their experiences of inpatient care

More information about their own and others' mental health problems:
'people stop being so nice, just like give me some leaflets, give me some information, not "hi, how are you" every single day, like I'd rather have some more information… about all different types of mental illness…'

Information about the rules and regulations of the unit:
'The dynamics of the relationships between myself and the nurses and the other patients was complicated because no-one knew what they were or were not allowed to do or say…'

Information about likely outcomes, or what to expect in the future:
'I'm still now getting told things like when I get better I'll be able to do this and that, which I would have liked maybe to know at the beginning when I was struggling, maybe I might have seen that as more of an aim, instead of more of a struggle.'

Other types of help that may be available, including help with benefits:
'I would have liked to have been told what help there was available and like, where – if it was just here or if there was somewhere else, just to know a bit more about the services available.'

Source: Street & Svanberg (2003).

---

provision. The findings of this work again centre on the importance of the adequacy of information about mental health provision and of good communication from staff, and of the importance of choice and appropriate support. However, some more unexpected issues came to light through this study. These included various negative consequences of care being offered at home, causing pain to some young people who had to then live with the association of home being the setting for the fights, arguments and psychotic phenomena that they had experienced when unwell (Rani et al. 2009).

In a similar vein to *Where Next?* Rani et al. also found that the timing of when information about proposed treatment and care is shared was crucial. They noted that even if adequate information is given at the point of engagement, this may not be retained due to the emotional turmoil that the young person or family is experiencing. Some families also reported that the support they had been offered was not what they wanted, and others felt that staff had made assumptions and not listened to what they had said. In addition, some parents struggled to take significant amounts of time off work in order to care for their child at home. Sometimes, managing the risk of a seriously ill young person at home became too much, and a number of parents expressed relief when their son or daughter was admitted to hospital.

More positively, Rani and colleagues found that young people and parents found treatment at home was preferable to admission to hospital wherever this was possible.

Care and treatment at home meant that they could continue the routine of family life to a greater extent, and the young person could maintain their friends and school contacts more easily. Young people and parents also told researchers that they also valued not having to do a lot of travelling to and from hospital.

In conclusion, Rani et al. note that, overall, hospital was seen as a necessary last resort, that home-based treatment is sometimes a preferable alternative, and that parents wanted to know that admission was an option if things at home became too difficult. However, they also note that new models of respite care which are able to offer immediate, short term support as an alternative to hospital admission may warrant further consideration. Indeed, this was the subsequent focus of an evaluation of alternatives to inpatient care for children and young people with complex mental health needs (National Institute for Health Research 2008).

Tier 4 CAMHS self-evaluation and young people's feedback data

Unpublished feedback provided to the National Youth Advocacy Service (NYAS) by young people and parents using Tier 4 services indicates that for some children, young people, parents and carers, the intensive support offered by an experienced staff group can be truly life changing. The practical things that helped young people as reported through the NYAS feedback included:

- education or school provision which felt relaxed and safe, with young people being given a choice of work to do and not being forced to do work they were uncomfortable with;
- trips out of the unit which provided new experiences and learning;
- the acquisition of new skills such as first aid training;
- help and support offered by unit staff to take exams;
- having a nurse around to listen to them when they needed it;
- good facilities.

What was less favourably reported on through the NYAS feedback was:

- the mix of young people can sometimes be difficult to live with;
- restrictions such as not being able to visit the bedrooms of other young people or to leave the building when they wanted;
- sleeping away from home and family;
- not having as many visitors as they would have liked.

Some views from parents were also provided. These indicated how frightening parents can find the admission of their child to a CAMHS unit. Things rated positively by parents included the thoroughness of assessments and the high staff to child ratio and support offered within unit schools.

Box 10.2 summarises some of the views about what makes a good inpatient unit as reported by young people as part of the *Where Next?* study (Street & Svanberg 2003).

BOX 10.2   What makes a good inpatient unit?: summary of views from young people

Pre-admission
- clear communication across services in the community;
- clear communication between community and inpatient or specialist services;
- clear information about sources of help and about mental health problems.

Admission
- services that are accessible;
- good quality and detailed information available about the service and about what to expect;
- consent to treatment is gained in a meaningful way;
- extra support is offered during the first few days of care and treatment and whilst children and young people become familiar with the service.

During stay
- clear information is provided about treatment and care, including roles of different members of staff, rules of the service and boundaries of acceptable behaviour;
- there is an ongoing dialogue between staff, young people and parents to promote involvement in their care and treatment as appropriate;
- staff are approachable, accessible and available to give support as and when needed;
- a range of individual and group-based therapeutic activities are on offer;
- the service is age-appropriate;
- education is available and is well supported;
- the environment is welcoming, homely, comfortable, clean, and ideally with gender segregated areas and space which addresses both privacy and safety needs of the young people.

Discharge
- children and young people, parents and carers are involved in discharge planning;
- close working with outside agencies is promoted to ensure a smooth handover, with graduated supported to promote reintegration back in to the community;
- joint working across health and other agencies is undertaken to address children and young people's varying needs, and in particular, to ensure that the needs of children and young people not returning home are fully addressed.

Source: Street and Svanberg (2003).

Delivering Tier 4 services in the future – some concluding messages

A number of recurring messages stand out from the range of material summarised in this chapter. It is clear that whilst over the last 10 years at least, there has been a widespread shift away from hospital inpatient care towards all sorts of health service provision, including CAMHS, being delivered on a community basis, Tier 4 inpatient care continues to play a vital role in supporting a significant number of children and young people. This includes those who may have complex mental health problems including co-morbid difficulties; those who present with highly risky behaviour; and those where family stresses are such that the 'safe space' away from home provided by an inpatient unit can be invaluable.

A clear message from service users is about having access to high quality information. This is in relation to when they will be admitted, for what reason and by whom – not least because, as a number of young people have graphically described, they are often scared at the prospect of being admitted to an inpatient unit. In a variety of consultations and research studies, children and young people have repeatedly highlighted the need for Tier 4 services to be accessible, flexible and to offer a homely age-appropriate environment where social activities and education sessions are provided and where the need for privacy is respected. Not being too far away from the child or young person's home is important so that family and peer relationships and contact can be maintained, and, above all, units must be able to respond promptly. These issues were prominent in the YoungMinds *Where Next?* study published nearly a decade ago and remain key challenges for the future development and delivery of this important area of CAMHS provision.

Meaningful participation is crucial if more people are to have a positive experience of help and support. Strengthening participation is consistent with the current government's principle of 'no decision about me without me' which is at the heart of liberating the NHS. However, there is still much we need to do to put children and young people centre stage in mental health policy, planning and service delivery.

References

Boylan, P. (2004). Children's Voices Project: feedback from children and young people about their experience and expectations of healthcare. London: Commission for Health Improvement (www.chi.nhs.uk/childrens_voices/Report.pdf).

Brady, M. (2009). Hospitalised children's views of the good nurse. *Nursing Ethics*, 16(5), 543–560.

Buston, K. (2002). Adolescents with mental health problems: what do they say about mental health services? *Journal of Adolescence*, 25(2), 231–242.

Day, C. (2008). Children's and young people's involvement and participation in mental health care. *Child and Adolescent Mental Health*, 13(1), 2–8.

Department for Children, Schools and Families. (2008). *Children and Young People's Workforce Strategy*. London: HMSO.

Department for Children, Schools and Families & Department of Health. (2008). *Children and Young People in Mind: the final report of the National CAMHS Review*. London: HMSO.

Department of Health. (2004). *National Service Framework for Children, Young People and Maternity Services*. London: HMSO.

Dogra, N. (2005). What do children and young people want from mental health services? *Current Opinion in Psychiatry*, 18, 370–373.

Farnfield, S. & Kaznap, M. (1998). What makes a helpful grown up?: children's views of professionals in mental health services. *Health Informatics Journal*, 4, 3–14.

Gibson, R. & Possamai, A. (2002). What young people think about CAMHS. *Clinical Psychology*, 18, 20–24.

Hovish, K., Weaver, T., Islam, Z., Paul, M. & Singh, S. (2012). Transition experiences of mental health service users, parents and professionals in the United Kingdom: a qualitative study. *Psychiatric Rehabilitation Journal*, 35, 251–257.

Lavis, P. and Hewson, L. (2011). *How Many Times So We Have To Tell You? A briefing from the National Advisory Council about what young people think about mental health and mental health services*. London: HMSO.

McDougall, T. & Bodley-Scott, S. (2008). Too much too young: under 18s on adult mental health wards. *Mental Health Practice*, 11(6), 12–15.

Main, L. (2006). *The Future of Mental Health: a vision for 2015 London*. London: The Sainsbury Centre for Mental Health.

Manteuffel, B., Stephoen, R., Sondheimer, D. & Fisher, S. (2008). Characteristics, service experiences and outcomes of transition aged youth in systems of care: programmatic and policy implications. *Journal of Behavioral Health Services and Research*, 35(4), 469–487.

Munoz-Solomando, A., Townley, M. & Williams, R. (2010). Improving transitions for young people who move from child and adolescent mental health services to mental health services for adults: lessons from research and young people's and practitioners' experiences. *Current Opinion in Psychiatry*, 23, 311–317.

National Institute for Health Research. (2008). *Alternatives to Inpatient Care for Children and Adolescents with Complex Mental Health Needs*. London: NIHR.

National Institute for Mental Health in England. (2009). *The Legal Aspects of Care and Treatment for Children and Young People with Mental Disorder: a guide for professionals*. London: NIMHE.

Office of the Children's Commissioner. (2007). *Pushed into the Shadows: young people's experience of adult mental health facilities*. London: OCC.

Paul, M. (2004). Decision making about children's mental health care: ethical challenges. *Advances in Psychiatric Treatment*, 10, 301–311.

Rani, J., Prosser, A., Worrall-Davies, A., Kiernan, K. & Hewson, L. (2009). User and carer views of CAMHS intensive home treatment services in Bradford. *Practice Development in Health Care*. doi:10.1002/pdh.292.

Robinson, S. (2010). Children and young people's views of health professionals in England. *Journal of Child Health Care*, 14(4), 310–326.

Sherman-Jones, A. (2003). Young people's perceptions of and access to health advice. *Nursing Times*, 99(30), 30–33.

Sinclair, R. (2004). Participation in practice: making it meaningful, effective and sustainable. *Children and Society*, 18, 106–118.

Singh, S.P. et al. (2009). *Transition from CAMHS to Adult Mental Health Services (TRACK): a study of policies, process and user and carer perspectives*. Executive Summary for the National Coordinating Centre for NHS Service Delivery and Organisation R+D (NCCSDO). London: NIHR.

Street, C. (2004). *Mental Health Services – What Children and Young People Want. Highlight 210*. London: National Children's Bureau.

Street, C. & Svanberg, J. (2003). *Where Next? New directions in inpatient mental health services for young people. Report 1: different models of provision for young people: facts and figures*. London: YoungMinds.

Worrall-Davies, A. (2008). Barriers and facilitators to children's and young people's views affecting CAMHS planning and delivery. *Child and Adolescent Mental Health*, 13(1), 16–18.

11

TRANSITION SERVICES

Tim McDougall

Key points

- Transition from adolescent to adult services is consistently experienced by young people as a major obstacle. Children and young people in contact with mental health services face two important transitions. First are those based on their age, and second are those based on their needs.
- Service-based transitions often lead to gaps in access for young people, particularly those aged 16 and 17. In some areas responsibility for leadership and delivery of services for young people aged 16 to 18 remains unclear, even within organisations providing lifespan mental health services.
- Some groups of children and young people face additional problems during transition which place them at added risk. These include young people with ADHD, those with autism spectrum disorders, young people with emerging personality disorder, looked after children and young people with learning disabilities. In some cases, young people are too old for CAMHS or not ill enough for adult mental health services (AMHS).
- The result of poorly developed transition services is that sometimes young people are left with no help when they need it and have no one to turn to in a crisis. The gains made from contact with CAMHS may be diminished or lost as a result of inadequate or failed transition to adult services. A number of service reviews confirm a lack of jointly agreed transition protocols.
- There is an urgent need to improve the transfer of care from CAMHS to adult services and the transitional care that supports this handover of care, for example from education and social care. Regardless of which service a young person may be moving to, professionals should get to know them before the transition, and plans should be in place to ensure that the transition is as smooth and as seamless as possible.

Introduction

It has been suggested that the transition to adulthood is becoming more complex, longer and more risky. It is a time when young people enter a new and exciting world with new rights and responsibilities. It is also the time when they take decisions that will affect the rest of their lives (Social Exclusion Unit 2005).

Some groups of children and young people face particular problems during transition which place them at increased risk. These include young people with emerging personality disorder; those with developmental disorders such as ADHD or autism spectrum condition (ASC); looked after children; and young people with learning disabilities.

Transition has been identified as a problem of long-standing concern for children and young people, their parents and carers, practitioners and policymakers. This is both in the UK and abroad (Davies 2003; McMillen & Raghavan 2009; Social Care Institute for Excellence 2011).

What do we mean by transition?

The Oxford Online Dictionary defines transition as 'a process or period of changing from one thing to another'. Transitions affect children and young people in contact with mental health services in a number of ways. First, they encounter transitions based on their age; and second, they face transitions due to their needs.

For many young people, the quality of the service they receive is affected by both their age *and* their needs. Children and young people are also affected by unplanned transitions and changes such as family breakdown and bereavement which are well known to have an affect on mental health and psychological well-being (DCSF 2008).

In their 'transitions toolkit', the government defines transition as a purposeful, planned process that addresses the medical, psychosocial, educational and vocational needs of adolescents and young adults with chronic physical and medical conditions as they move from child centred to adult oriented healthcare systems (Department of Health 2006).

CAMHS have historically been planned, commissioned and delivered as part of children's services. To a greater or lesser extent this has enabled links with universal and targeted services for children and young people. However, it has also meant that in some areas specialist mental health services for children and young people and adults have been planned, commissioned and delivered separately. This of course is problematic when young people need to transition from one service to the next, which is usually when they reach 16 or 18 years of age.

What does national policy and guidance tell us?

The need for robust transition planning between CAMHS and AMHS was highlighted as far back as 1999 when the *National Service Framework for Mental Health* was published (Department of Health 1999). This was supported by a key performance indicator set by the Healthcare Commission and the recommendations of the Children's Safeguarding Review published in 2002. Over a decade on, many NHS trusts still do not have dedicated transition protocols (DCSF 2008) and the latest government's strategy to improve mental health (Department of Health 2011) repeats the policy messages announced over a decade earlier to improve transition services. *No Health without Mental Health* states that service transition from CAMHS to adult mental health can be improved by early planning, listening to young people, providing appropriate and accessible information, and focusing on joint commissioning and outcomes (Department of Health 2011). Guidance for mental health and social care commissioners has been produced which focuses on young people making the transition from child and adolescent to adult services (National Mental Health Delivery Unit 2011; Joint Commissioning Panel for Mental Health 2012).

The *National Service Framework for Children, Young People and Maternity Services* (Department of Health 2004a) includes a standard on mental health which includes good practice markers in relation to transition. However, broader NSF guidance on transition for children moving to adult health services excludes mental health (Department of Health 2006). It does say, however, that all young people should have access to age appropriate services which are responsive to their specific needs as they grow into adulthood (Department of Health 2004a).

Despite a suite of national policy and associated guidance, several reviews and evaluations all confirm a lack of jointly agreed planning for transition within mental health and partner services (DCSF 2008; Singh et al. 2009). A review of Tier 4 CAMHS commissioned by the Department of Health found that young people's transition needs are generally unmet by specialist CAMHS (Department of Health 2009). The recent guidance published by the Joint Commissioning Panel for Mental Health (2012) suggests that formal working arrangements should be put in place to address structural and procedural difficulties arising from the interface of CAMHS and AMHS and the differences in culture across the two services.

In his review of children's services for the Department of Health Professor Ian Kennedy points out that the transition of care is a phenomenon created by professionals and the structures within which they work. He suggests that a young person's needs and the care they require to meet them evolve, yet services often change abruptly when children reach the arbitrary age of 16 or 18 (Department of Health 2010). Amongst other things, the Kennedy Report recommended that Government should map out responsibility for the care of children and adults in order to expose the problem of transition (Department of Health 2010).

What is the scale of the problem?

The majority of mental illness starts in the teenage years (Kim-Cohen et al. 2003), which is precisely when most child and adolescent services stop and adult services start. In some areas of the UK dedicated services are available for children from birth to 18. In other areas they 'cut off' at 16 and responsibility for 17-year-olds lies with adult services. In some areas this works well, and in others the responsibility for leadership and delivery of services for young people aged 16 to 18 is unclear, even within organisations providing lifespan mental health services.

However, the Audit Commission (1999) report, *Children in Mind* found that less than a quarter of health authorities had specified transfer arrangements from CAMHS to adult services. This finding was supported by the Mental Health Foundation (Singh et al. 2005) who reported no clarity or agreement as to the age at which CAMHS ends. Nearly a decade on there continues to be no standardised model of service delivery for CAMHS. There are dedicated 16–19 teams in some parts of the UK but these are not generally available. In some places, access is determined by whether the young person is in school.

The National CAMHS Review suggested that chronological age is not the best determinant for service provision, and instead recommended that services should be based on individual needs (DCSF 2008). This was supported in the Department of Health (2010) Kennedy Report which suggested that although the division of funding for children's and adult's services may be bureaucratically convenient it often makes no sense at all to the young people concerned. Instead, Kennedy suggested, young people should be able to enjoy a continuity of care that ignores birthdays and focuses on needs (Department of Health 2010).

The situation is no clearer across wider children's services. Local authority children's services including schools, colleges and youth services are generally provided up to the age of 19, although some young people with disabilities can receive services until they are 25. Similarly, children in care can access support from their local authority up until the age of 21, or 25 if they are engaged in a programme of education or training. Youth justice services work with children and young people between 10 and 17. The impact of this variability is that some people are unable to access services due to their age, needs or postcode.

What does research and good practice tell us?

In addition to policy declarations a number of transition 'toolkits' have been published. These are designed to support service providers and commissioners deliver better transition support to children and young people including those leaving inpatient services (Health and Social Care Advisory Service 2005; National Children's Bureau 2008). However, these too have not generally helped enable comprehensive improvements in the experience of transition for young people.

There have been several large scale studies of transitional support for young people in contact with mental health services. The largest of these was the Department of Health funded *Transition from CAMHS to Adult Mental Health Services (TRACK)* study across several NHS trusts in Greater London and the West Midlands (Singh et al. 2009). This looked at service organisation, policies, and transition protocols, and included a focus on users' and carers' experiences of transition from CAMHS to AMHS. By tracking care pathways, interviewing service users and exploring outcomes, the TRACK study identified factors that enhance and impede effective transition. The TRACK study showed that:

1   there was a lack of transition protocols in the study areas;
2   age-based transition boundaries varied from 16 to 21 years and over, with 18 being most common;
3   protocols were based on policy documents, but differed on practical aspects of transition;
4   most protocols identified the service user as central to the transition process, yet none specified ways of preparing them for transition;
5   three-quarters of the protocols had no provision for ensuring continuity of care for young people who were not accepted by adult services.

The TRACK study came to several important conclusions. For the vast majority of service users it was clear that transition was poorly organised, badly managed and a negative experience for young people. The researchers claimed that this was partly due to mutual misconceptions between CAMHS and AMHS leading to structural and ideological obstacles getting in the way of good transitional care. This, they suggested, accentuated the barriers that pre-existed between CAMHS and AMHS. The report of the TRACK study for the Department of Health made recommendations about how services should be planned, configured and delivered to ensure good continuity of care (Singh et al. 2009).

The Mental Health Foundation's 'Listen Up!' project (2007) makes the case for fundamental change in the basic service model for young people. It calls on commissioners to designate a lead agency and person to coordinate the commissioning of services for young people aged 16–25. It also calls for the provision of long term funding to voluntary sector organisations, and for statutory youth mental health services in general to learn from the voluntary sector's example of person-centred provision. The report is primarily aimed at those who commission and fund services for children and young people, as well as those working within the voluntary and community sectors and statutory sector who are setting up or developing services for young people with mental health and emotional problems.

What does the law tell us?

The need to ensure that children and young people experience good transitional care is supported by mental health and children's legislation.

The law affecting transition has evolved in recent years. A key milestone was the National Health Service Act which came into force in 2006. This required the government to ensure that people had access to a comprehensive health service focusing on the prevention, diagnosis and treatment of illness. This was to involve hospital services and facilities for the prevention of illness, care of people who are ill and aftercare for those who had suffered from illness (HM Government 2006). Duties were delegated to NHS trusts to commission and provide health services for local populations. The NHS Act has now been superseded by the Health and Social Care Bill which passed through the final parliamentary stages as this book was being written.

What do children and young people tell us?

Transition is consistently experienced by children and young people as a major obstacle in their recovery (DCSF 2008; YoungMinds 2005). Their views have been clearly articulated through a range of nationally commissioned projects and engagement events. These include YoungMInds *Stressed out and Struggling* focus group report (YoungMinds 2005) and the report on transition commissioned by the National Advisory Council for Children's Mental Health and Psychological Wellbeing (DCSF 2008).

In a research briefing Brodie and colleagues (2011) point out that young people, their families and carers want their views to be taken seriously and to participate actively in the process of transition. They value good information, consistent support from a key worker and flexible, non-stigmatising community-based services appropriate for their age group.

A study by the National Children's Bureau (2008) focused specifically on young people leaving inpatient services. They told researchers that it was important to know who was leading their care on discharge so that CAMHS can hand over the baton of care and responsibility. Young people reported a range of obstacles to this happening in practice, including large caseloads, uncertainty about responsibility for aftercare and problems with funding. They talked about being disappointed by aftercare plans that collapsed, and feeling let down when promises about placements didn't come to fruition. Young people's views about hospital, community and home-based services in general are discussed further in Chapter 10.

Children and young people in vulnerable groups

Various writers have highlighted the risks of poor transition in particular groups of children and young people (Richards and Vostanis 2004; Maughan 2005). The success of Early Intervention in Psychosis (EIP) services in supporting young people to stay well and to remain in education, training or employment is a good example of successful service delivery specifically aimed at adolescents and young adults in transition. Young people are able to access age and developmentally appropriate care. However, this model has not been tested with other disorders.

The impact of poorly planned and developed transition services is that young people may be left with no help at a time when research suggests they may need it most. Sometimes the positive therapeutic benefit they have gained whilst in the care of CAMHS is diminished or lost as they transition to adult services.

Research from the third sector by charities such as YoungMinds, Rethink and the Mental Health Foundation has highlighted that young people sometimes find adult services inaccessible, inflexible and unable to meet their needs. Some children and young people are more vulnerable to poor transition due to their complex or additional needs. These include:

1   looked after children;
2   children and young people with learning disabilities and mental health difficulties;
3   children and young adults with ADHD;
4   young people with ASCs;
5   16- and 17-year-olds;
6   young offenders.

Looked after children

Children in the care of local authorities are at five-fold risk of mental disorder (Green et al. 2005) and risk of suicide as adults (Vinnerljung et al. 2006).

Children and young people with learning disabilities

Children and young people with learning disabilities are over six times more likely than children in general to develop mental disorder (Emerson & Hatton 2007). The difficulties they face with transition have been well documented and have been the focus of a government support programme (Department for Children, Schools and Families 2007). *Aiming High for Disabled Children* (Department for Education 2007) highlights the need for responsive, coordinated and timely services which are easily accessible at key transition points.

Fraser (2005) reported the existence of geographical variation in acceptance criteria among community support teams and learning disabilities services. Some teams only support children and young people with severe learning disabilities, whereas others will include those with more mild difficulties. There is also disagreement on what constitutes 'challenging behaviour' and thus on the level of support that should be provided.

Lamb and colleagues (2008) suggest that learning disability services often have good links and effective transfer of care to adult learning disability services. Problems are more likely to arise, they suggest, in relation to young people with mild or moderate learning disability and a low level of general functioning and for those with higher functioning ASCs, particularly when there is no clear cut co-morbid psychiatric disorder.

Transition from CAMHS services, particularly for young people with less severe learning disabilities, is an area of concern. In some areas young people become the responsibility of learning disability services when they become 16. However, this applies primarily to young people with more severe disorders. For those with more high functioning conditions such as Asperger's syndrome or mild autistic spectrum disorders, responsibility for local service provision tends to be less clear (Fraser 2005).

ADHD

ADHD is no longer recognised exclusively as a disorder of childhood. Approximately 15 per cent of children with this condition will have ongoing impairment into adulthood (NICE 2008). Many young people with ADHD make the transition from childhood to adulthood smoothly whereas others struggle as they encounter problems with hyperactivity and inattention in higher education, employment or adult relationships (Willoughby 2003).

Children and young people diagnosed with ADHD as children often require transition to AMHS. However, the provision of adult ADHD services is limited in the UK and most young adults are unable to access appropriate specialist services (Asherson 2005; Nutt et al. 2007). AMHS provide assessment and treatment interventions for adults with a range of mental health problems. Some of these can appear similar to ADHD, particularly bipolar disorder and personality disorders, and, to varying degrees, each of these disorders involves difficulties with activity, behaviour regulation, impulsiveness and inattention. Many adult mental health professionals will not have encountered ADHD and some may lack the knowledge skills and expertise to support an adult service user with ADHD. This makes the potential for misdiagnosis and inappropriate treatment high (Ryan & McDougall 2008).

Where adult services do exist, the evidence from young people is that the transition process is not usually a positive event and is associated with significant concerns and anxieties (Willoughby 2003; Beresford 2004). Various reports have confirmed that transitional arrangements for young people with ADHD are often poor, lack strategy and are frequently managed on a case to case basis (NHS Quality Improvement Scotland 2007).

It is not only transitions from CAMHS to AMHS that young people with ADHD may struggle with. There is evidence that the transitions from junior school to secondary school, and the process of leaving college to start employment can also be stressful (While et al. 2004; Horstmann & Steer 2007). Access to one to one teacher support may decrease, and the demands generated by a bigger peer group may increase. For children with ADHD, the challenges may be greater due to deficits in organising, planning and memory skills which are essential to manage this transition smoothly (Ryan & McDougall 2008). It is therefore essential that health professionals support young people with ADHD to navigate transitions successfully. NICE (2008) guidance addresses both the transition of care and treatment recommendations for young people transitioning to adulthood and it has been suggested that this model may be helpful for other groups of young people, including those on the autism spectrum (DCSF 2008).

ASCs

The difficulties of young people with ASC often become evident during periods of transition when change produces additional disruption to routines and access to familiar faces.

In a report on mental health transitions for young people the Social Care Institute for Excellence (2011) point out that AMHS are generally very poor for people with ASCs.

Young people aged 16 and 17

Young people aged 16 who require hospital admission for the treatment of their mental disorder have historically had poor access to services. In some areas of the UK the responsibility for leadership and delivery of services for young people aged 16 to 18 has frequently been unclear, even within organisations providing lifespan mental health services.

Section 31 of the Mental Health Act 2007 inserts a new provision (section 131A) into the Mental Health Act 1983. This applies to patients under the age of 18 who are liable to be detained in hospital under the 1983 Act, or are admitted to hospital as informal patients under section 131 of the 1983 Act. Section 31 imposes a duty on commissioners to ensure that age appropriate inpatient services are available, and a duty on hospital managers to ensure the environment of such patients is suitable having regard to their age, subject to their needs. Since this amendment to the Mental Health Act has been made there have been fewer inappropriate admissions to adult mental health wards in England. However, in some areas there remains a shortage of suitable hospital beds for 16 and 17 year olds and considerable weaknesses in transition arrangements for young people moving to adult services.

Young offenders

Care, support and transition needs of young people with a mental disorder who pose a risk to others or have a forensic history are complex. Differences in eligibility criteria can result in gaps in access to services or treatment in settings that do not meet the young person's developmental needs (Lamb et al. 2008). Young people in custody have increased risk of mental disorders and are at heightened risk of suicide (Youth Justice Board for England and Wales 2005). Their needs are discussed further in Chapter 9.

Summary

Young people aged 16 and 17 are making the transition to adulthood, and so may have a range of needs including those related to living independently and developing as young adults. Partnerships should be monitored to ensure that joint strategic planning is in place and that the full range of partners are playing their part in improving outcomes for children and young people during transition. However, monitoring in itself is not sufficient to ensure that children's and young people's mental health is improved. Instead, evidence should be required to show that improvements in service commissioning are reflected in improvements on the ground.

Robust transition planning offers a real window of opportunity for change. Whilst the *National Service Framework for Mental Health* required all organisations to have a transition policy in place, not all providers of CAMHS and AMHS have protocols in place. For local partners, joint strategic needs assessments, robust children and young people's plans and integrated commissioning arrangements also present an opportunity to improve outcomes for young people. These should focus on the full range of needs including those related to mental health and psychological well-being.

There is an urgent need to improve the transfer of care from CAMHS to AMHS and the transitional care that supports these transitions, for example from education and social care. For NHS partners, a stronger focus on transitions may help to improve pathways between CAMHS and AMHS. Regardless of which service a young person may be moving to, professionals should get to know them before the transition, and plans should be in place to ensure that the transition is as smooth and as seamless as possible.

References

Asherson, P. (2005). Clinical assessment and treatment of attention deficit hyperactivity disorder in adults. *Expert Review of Neurotherapeutics*, 5(4), 525–539.

Audit Commission. (1999). *Children in Mind: child and adolescent mental health services*. London: Audit Commission.

Beresford, B. (2004). On the road to nowhere? Young disabled people and transition. *Child: Health Care and Development*, 30(6), 581–587.

Brodie, I., Chapman, R. & Clapton, J. (2011). *Mental Health Service Transitions for Young People*, Research Briefing 37, London: Social Care Institute for Excellence.

Clark, A., O'Malley, A. & Woodham. (2005). Children with complex mental health problems: needs, costs and predictors over 1 year. *Child and Adolescent Mental Health*, 10(4), 170–178.

Davies, M. (2003). Addressing the needs of youth in transition to adult. *Administration and Policy in Mental Health*, 30(6), 495–509.

Department for Children, Schools and Families. (2007). *A Transition Guide for all Services: key information for professionals about the transition process for disabled young people*. London: HMSO.

Department for Children, Schools and Families & Department of Health. (2008) *Children and Young People in Mind: the final report of the National CAMHS Review*. London: HMSO.

Department for Education. (2007.) *Aiming High for Disabled Children: better support for families*. London: HMSO.

Department of Health. (1999). *National Service Framework for Mental Heath*. London: HMSO.

Department of Health. (2004). *National Service Framework for Mental Health*. London: HMSO.

Department of Health. (2006). *Transition: getting it right for children and young people – improving the transition of children with long term conditions to adult services*. London: HMSO.

Department of Health. (2009). *The Evidence Base to Guide Development of Tier 4 CAMHS*. London: HMSO.

Department of Health. (2010). *Getting it Right for Children and Young People: overcoming cultural barriers in the NHS so as to meet their needs* (The Kennedy Report). London: HMSO.

Department of Health. (2011). *No Health without Mental Health: a cross government mental health outcomes strategy for people of all ages*. London: HMSO.

Emerson, M. & Hatton, C. (2007). Mental health of children and adolescents with intellectual disabilities in Britain. *British Journal of Psychiatry*, 191, 493–499.

Fraser, W. (2005). Children and adolescents who have a learning disability: the challenges to services. In: Williams, R. & Kerfoot, M. (eds). *Child and Adolescent Mental Health Services: strategy, planning, delivery, and evaluation*. London: Oxford University Press.

Green, H., McGinnity, A., Meltzer, H., Ford, T. & Goodman, R. (2005). *Mental Health of Children and Young People in Great Britain*. London: ONS.

Health and Social Care Advisory Service. (2005). *CAMHS to Adult Transition*. London: HASCAS.

HM Government. (2006). *National Health Service Act*. London: HMSO.

Horstmann, K. & Steer, J. (2007). Transition into a secondary school for children with a diagnosis of attention deficit hyperactivity disorder or autistic spectrum disorder: a pilot group. *Clinical Psychology Forum*, 176, 14–17.

Joint Commissioning Panel for Mental Health. (2012). *Guidance for Commissioners of Mental Health Services for Young People Making the Transition for Child and Adolescent to Adult Services: volume 2: practical mental health commissioning*. London: Raffertys.

Kim-Cohen, J., Caspi, A. & Moffitt, T. (2003). Prior juvenile diagnoses in adults with mental disorder: developmental follow-back of a prospective longitudinal cohort. *Archives of General Psychiatry*, 60, 709–717.

Lamb, C., Hall, D., Kelvin, R. & van Beinum, M. (2008). *Working at the CAMHS/Adult Interface: good practice guidance for the provision of psychiatric services to adolescents/young adults*. A joint paper from the Interfaculty working group of the Child and Adolescent Faculty and the General and Community Faculty of the Royal College of Psychiatrists. London: RCP.

McDougall, T., Worrall-Davies, A., Hewson, L., Richardson, G. & Cotgrove, A. (2008). Tier 4 Child and Adolescent Mental Health Services: inpatient care, day services and alternatives: an overview of Tier 4 CAMHS provision in the UK. *Child and Adolescent Mental Health*, 13(4), 173–180.

McMillen, J. & Raghavan, R. (2009). Pediatric to adult mental health service use of young people leaving the foster care system. *Journal of Adolescent Health*, 44(1), 7–13.

Maughan, B. (2005). Continuities between childhood and adult life. *British Journal of Psychiatry*, 187, 301–303.

National Children's Bureau. (2008). *Managing the Transitions from Adolescent Psychiatric Inpatient Care*. London: NCB.

National Mental Health Delivery Unit. (2011). *Planning Mental Health Services for Young Adults: improving transition: a resource for health and social care commissioners*. London: NMHDU.

NHS Quality Improvement Scotland. (2007). *ADHD: services over Scotland: report of the service profiling exercise 2007*. Edinburgh: NHS Scotland.

NICE. (2008). *Attention Deficit Hyperactivity Disorder: diagnosis and management of ADHD in children, young people and adults*. London: NCCMH.

Nutt, D., Fone, K., Asherson, P., Bramble, D., Hill, P., Matthews, K., Morris, K., Santosh, P., Sonuga-Barke, E., Taylor, E., Weiss, M. & Young, S. (2007). Evidence-based guidelines for management of attention deficit hyperactivity disorder in adolescents in transition to adult services and in adults: recommendations from the British Association for Psychopharmacology. *Journal of Psychopharmacology*, 21(1), 10–41.

Richards, M. & Vostanis, P. (2004). Interprofessional perspectives on transitional mental health services for young people aged 16-19 years. *Journal of Interprofessional Care*, 18(20), 115–128.

Ryan, N. & McDougall, T. (2008). *Nursing Children and Young People with ADHD*. London: Routledge.

Singh, S.P., Evans, N., Sireling, L. & Stuart, H. (2005) Mind the gap: the interface between child and adult mental health services. *Psychiatric Bulletin* 29, 292–294.

Singh, S., Moli, P., Islam, Z. et al. (2009). *Transition from CAMHS to Adult Mental Health Services (TRACK): a study of service organisation, policies, process and user and carer perspectives*. Executive Summary for the National Coordinating Centre for NHS Service Delivery and Organisation R+D (NCCSDO). London: NCCSDO.

Social Care Institute for Excellence. (2011). *Mental Health Service Transitions for Young People*. London: SCIE.

Social Exclusion Unit. (2005). *Transitions: young adults with complex needs*. London: HMSO.

Vinnerljung, B., Hjern, A. & Lindblad, F. (2006). Suicide attempts and severe psychiatric morbidity among former child welfare clients: a national cohort study. *Journal of Child Psychology and Psychiatry*, 47(7), 723–733.

While, A., Forbes, A. & Fullman, R. (2004). Good practices that address continuity during transition from child to adult care: syntheses of the evidence. *Child: Health Care and Development*, 30(5), 439–452.

Willoughby, M. (2003). Developmental course of ADHD symptomatology during the transition from childhood to adolescence: a review with recommendations. *Journal of Child Psychology and Psychiatry*, 44(1), 88–106.

YoungMinds. (2005). *Stressed Out and Struggling*. London: YoungMinds.

Youth Justice Board for England and Wales. (2005). *Mental Health Needs and Provision*. London: YJB.

12

COMMISSIONING

Marie Crofts and Helen Hipkiss

Key points

- For commissioning of Tier 4 services to be successful it is essential that all partners have the same understanding of what commissioning is. Commissioning can be defined as the process of specifying, securing and monitoring services to meet people's needs at a strategic level. This applies to all services, whether they are provided by the local authority, the NHS, other public agencies or by the private or voluntary sectors.
- A national analysis of Tier 4 service reviews found that there was enormous inconsistency and variability in terms of access, availability and levels of care for children and young people, and that the data required to strategically commission services was at best patchy and at worst non-existent.
- Tier 4 CAMHS commissioning is expected to be strategic, underpinned by evidence, based on the needs of children and young people and focused on outcomes. In some parts of the UK Tier 4 commissioning is none of these things. Instead, children and young people requiring hospital, intensive community and home-based services can not access the support that they need and that we know to be effective. This not only compromises their life chances, but it is also hugely expensive for health and local authority commissioners.
- In 2010 the government set out the future arrangements for commissioning NHS services in England. In 2013 the National Commissioning Board became responsible for commissioning specialised services including hospital, as well as some intensive community and home-based services.
- Clinical Commissioning Groups also need to understand specialised services when commissioning local services to ensure that children and young people move across the pathway in a seamless manner. Similarly, local health and wellbeing boards (HWBs) play a role in ensuring services are commissioned across a pathway that is from community services right through to complex specialised Tier 4 services. They have statutory responsibilities and bring together the key strategic partners in each area.

Introduction

This chapter is aimed at both CAMHS commissioners and providers. It explores the process of commissioning Tier 4 services in an integrated pathway with other CAMHS services. The principles of joint planning and commissioning are used to set out a framework for commissioning specialised CAMHS and the process carried out by one regional specialised commissioning team is given as an example. The roles of the new commissioning organisations within England, including NHS England, are explored.

What is commissioning?

For commissioning of Tier 4 services to be successful it is essential that all partners have the same understanding of what commissioning is. Commissioning can be defined as 'the process of specifying, securing and monitoring services to meet people's needs at a strategic level. This applies to all services, whether they are provided by the local authority, the NHS, other public agencies or by the private or voluntary sectors' (Audit Commission, 2003).

Background and context

Commissioning specialist treatment and care which is of high cost and low volume requires specific knowledge and skills and needs robust procedures in place to ensure effective delivery. Although children and young people needing inpatient and other specialist care for mental health problems fall into this bracket, a robust mechanism for commissioning such services is still variable across the country. Where more standardised and quality assured processes are more apparent they may not be able to adjust and flex in a way which meets the changing needs of young people in a timely manner.

The National CAMHS Support Service (NCSS) in their publication *Better Mental Health Outcomes for Children and Young People: A resource directory for commissioners* (2011) stated that 'The Government's mental health strategy is clear that high quality services depend on high quality commissioning.' It suggests that too often the commissioning of mental health services has not received sufficient attention at senior level, and there has been an inadequate focus on outcomes and the way that services can be commissioned to achieve better outcomes.

Commissioning specialist high quality mental health services can be particularly challenging because provision spans a wide range of agencies and settings across children's and adult services. In addition, mental health services cannot be commissioned in isolation to other service provision for children and young people with severe, complex or persistent mental disorders. This is a complex and complicated business at the multi-agency level of provision and only increases in complexity when attempting to commission highly specialised services for children and young people.

A national analysis of Tier 4 reviews (Kurtz 2007) revealed that there was enormous inconsistency and variability in terms of access, availability and levels of care for children and young people in England, but more worryingly the data available for local analysis and review on which to commission services was at best patchy and at worst non-existent.

In her review, Kurtz found weakness in the commissioning process across many English regions and, in some cases, an absence of effective provider and commissioner dialogue through which to reach agreement on the priorities for Tier 4 to address.

Commissioning for CAMHS pathways into Tier 4

Usual practice has been for specialist community CAMHS services (Tiers 2 and 3) to develop and expand through funding from the former CAMHS Grant. This saw the growth of community children and adolescent mental health services nationally. This growth, however, wasn't replicated within the NHS inpatient settings for young people, and remained inconsistent on a number of levels (O'Herlihy et al. 2007; Cotgrove et al. 2007), not least in terms of cost, treatment pathways and the quality of experience for young people using these services. In contrast to the NHS the independent sector providers expanded their share of the market considerably during this period.

The need for inpatient and other Tier 4 services cannot be defined by diagnosis or problems presented but by a level of need which cannot be met by local community services. This may vary across local CAMHS. This in itself makes the job of commissioning appropriate and standardised Tier 4 services more difficult.

Robust care pathways have been difficult to create for Tier 4 services as the criteria for referral into Tier 4 and for when inpatient treatment is required are variable across the country and even across individual services. As community CAMHS has grown at different paces and with different sets of criteria and flexibility to manage young people, the need for inpatient and other Tier 4 services has become hugely variable. Varying levels of admission are common and in some way dependent on the development of intensive home treatment or active management of high-risk young people in alternative ways to hospital admission.

The Joint Planning and Commissioning Cycle

The Joint Planning and Commissioning Cycle (Department for Education and Skills 2006) offers a framework for undertaking the commissioning of services across the NHS and local authorities. The joint process is useful for Tier 4 services as it enables commissioners to:

- promote an integrated approach to meeting population needs across health, education and social care;
- manage the relationship between needs and services;
- shift the balance between service tiers;
- manage the relationship with expanding private and voluntary sectors;
- reconfigure public services in the context of overall need.

Although in England the commissioning of Tier 4 services is becoming more clearly specified from 2013 (Department of Health 2012b) the steps outlined below are still relevant to ensure that Tier 4 services are appropriate to meet the needs of the local population and fit within a clear care pathway across all the tiers.

The cycle has nine steps (see Figure 12.1).

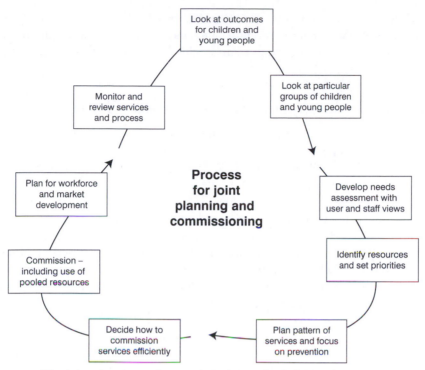

FIGURE 12.1   The joint planning and commissioning cycle (DfES 2006)

Step 1: look at outcomes for children and young people

The cycle starts with asking 'What outcomes will the service deliver for young people?' This enables the commissioner to consider what is needed for the client group rather than what services to put in place.

It is essential that commissioners contract for services that are safe and clinically effective by using best practice as defined, for example, by NICE. By designing services that are based on treatments and clinical pathways that are evidence-based, commissioners can be assured that they are achieving the best outcomes for the children and young people in the service. In addition, other service outcomes that need to be considered include:

- An appropriate balance of CAMHS Tier 3 and Tier 4 that more accurately delivers the range and types of service responses required based on the mental health needs of children and young people.
- A larger proportion of children and young people with severe and complex mental health needs will receive appropriate services through intensive non-bed-based CAMH services delivered in the family home.
- A significant reduction of children and young people inappropriately admitted to adult mental health services.
- Robust evaluations of the change in structure and provision of CAMHS Tier 3 and Tier 4 and the effectiveness of these changes.

As well as designing services based on practice for which there is an evidence of good outcomes, it is also important to monitor outcomes for the individuals who receive the service. This should be monitored in terms of clinical outcomes, patient rated outcomes and patient experience.

Step 2: look at particular groups of children and young people

The next step looks at which groups of children and young people Tier 4 services will be provided for. The challenge here is to think in broad terms. Referring to the local Children and Young People Plan will give some indications. Local staff as well as talking to young people will also help identify the groups.

The Royal College of Psychiatrists (2006) suggests that the commissioning of Tier 4 services should be underpinned by a comprehensive joint agency needs assessment to establish the range and capacity of Tier 4 services required in a given region. The three key agencies of health, education and social care must work in partnership along with significant others, including the youth justice system and housing organisations in order to achieve this. It should address needs across all tiers and include a prospective audit of CAMHS Tier 4 cases in the independent sector.

It should be recognised that national evidence shows that children with complex needs often have two or more disorders and a variety of risks which will affect an outcome (Rutter 1987). Tier 4 needs, therefore, to provide services for co-morbidities such as learning disability and mental health disorder and risks, which will often not fit into specific groupings. Commissioning must reflect this approach to ensure a flexible approach to meet needs, not just diagnosis.

Step 3: develop needs assessment with user and staff views

There is no need to reinvent the wheel. Much of the evidence of need is available from national epidemiological evidence. However, this will also need to link with local work completed in the CAMHS Strategy and Children and Young People Plan. It is important to ask users and staff their views. Examples given by young people of an improvement in patient experience/satisfaction include 'staff listen to me', 'when I needed help it happened quickly', 'I wanted my family to be able to visit me', 'I was able to go home with support' (Hipkiss 2011).

Organising local events where users and staff can discuss their concerns is a quick method of identifying local needs, which can then be reviewed alongside the formal needs assessment to identify gaps. The Child and Maternal Health Observatory (CHIMAT) offer a variety of tools to support needs assessment and links with Joint Strategic Needs Assessment, identifying the gaps needed to deliver appropriate levels of service to the local population. The commissioning should be based on a joint strategy and delivery based on the needs assessment of the population.

Step 4: identify resources and set priorities

Once the local needs have been assessed, there will be a need to identify the resources available and prioritise what the programme will deliver. As the service will impact across agencies it is useful to form a multi-agency group that can access various budgets to support the work. It is also helpful to reflect on the outcomes the service needs to deliver, as these will often be across agency outcomes that will support partnership working and funding.

There is a growing evidence base for CAMHS (National CAMHS Support Service 2011) and the economic case for Tier 4 services which work in an integrated manner with community teams (Knapp et al. 2011). Levers such as statutory guidance and policy frameworks will also guide local priorities. The former Care Services Improvement Partnership (CSIP 2010) published a resource for commissioning age-appropriate services for children and young people under 18 (see Table 12.1).

Step 5: plan pattern of service and focus on prevention

Putting together services at this stage can seem difficult especially as work will be across local, regional and national providers. However, there are examples described in other chapters that can be developed. Liaising with other commissioners and the providers will help develop a holistic service.

Key questions to address are:

- What is the definition of Tier 4? What are the criteria and thresholds for referral into Tier 4 CAMHS?
- What are the interventions known to be effective to meet the needs of the Tier 4 population?
- What will the elements of the service be?
- Are there non-bed-based alternatives to admission with as good or better outcomes?
- Who's going to deliver them?
- How will the service be delivered?
- Where will the service take place?
- What is the cost?
- What outcomes should be measured?
- How will the process and its impact on the outcomes for children be evaluated?
- What are the key deliverables or criteria for a successful service meeting the needs of children and young people?

Tier 4 service commissioners need to consider the whole CAMHS pathway. Developing highly specialised services that do not take into account the range of local provision may result in a disjointed service with no opportunities for step up or down facilities. A modern NHS expects services to be community-based with limited inpatient stays. Commissioning Tier 4 services that include outreach, support for local CAMHS teams, 24-hour access and a range of other specialist non-bed-based services will enable children and young people to stay at home wherever possible but be accessible at times of crisis or significant need.

TABLE 12.1 Resources for commissioning age-appropriate services for children and young people under 18

Title	Published by	Status
Stressed Out and Struggling: A Call to Action: commissioning mental health services for 16-25s	YoungMinds	Good practice
The Evidence Base to Guide Development of Tier 4 CAMHS	Department of Health / National CAMHS Support Service	Research and policy summary
CAMHS to Adult Transition: self assessment checklist	HASCAS	Self assessment checklist
CAMHS to Adult Transition: annotated bibliography	HASCAS	Transition research literature review
Managing the Transitions from Adolescent Psychiatric In-Patient Care	National Children's Bureau	Good practice toolkit
Tier 4 CAMHS: Improving, Expanding and Reforming	Department of Health / National CAMHS Support Service	Handbook
Implementing the Mental Health 2007: what boards need to know and do	The NHS Confederation	Briefing paper
The Legal Aspects of the Care and Treatment of Children and Young People with Mental Disorders	NIMHE	Professionals guidance
Working Together to Provide Age Appropriate Environments and Services for Mental Health Patients Aged Under 18: a briefing for commissioners of adult mental health services and CAMHS	National Mental Health Development Unit	Briefing
North West CAMHS Needs Assessment	NIMHE / CSIP	Commissioned report
Children and Young People on Adult Mental Health Wards in the North West	NHS North West / Cheshire and Merseyside Child Health Development Programme / CSIP	Commissioned report
Tier 4 CAMHS Admissions to NHS and Independent Sector Beds in the North West	NHS North West / CSIP	Commissioned report
Out of Area Placements of Young People Requiring Tier 4 CAMHS Admission in the North West	NHS North West / CSIP	Commissioned report
Transitions: young adults with complex needs	Office of the Deputy Prime Minister	Report

Title	Published by	Status
Out of the Shadows?: a review of the responses and recommendations made in Pushed Into the Shadows: young people's experience of adult mental health facilities	11 MILLION / YoungMinds	Report
Quality Network for Inpatient CAMHS / Quality Improvement Network for Multi Agency CAMHS: improving access to inpatient CAMHS and appropriate alternatives	QNIC / QINMAC / Royal College of Psychiatrists	Position statement
The Mental Health Act: essential information for parents and carers	RETHINK / NIMHE	Guidance
Safe and Appropriate Care for Young People on Adult Mental Health Wards	Royal College of Psychiatrists Centre for Quality Improvement / NIMHE / National Patient Safety Agency	Quality standards
Systematic Review and Mapping Study of Alternatives to Inpatient Care for Children and Adolescents with Complex Mental Health Needs	National Institute for Health Research Service Delivery and Organisation Programme	Report
Regional Reviews of Tier 4 Child and Adolescent Mental Health Services	CSIP / National CAMHS Support Service	Report
Tier 4 CAMHS: Inpatient Care, Day Services and Alternatives: an overview of Tier 4 CAMHS provision in the UK	Journal of Child and Adolescent Mental Health	Paper
Young People on Adult Mental Health Wards	Mental Health Practice	Paper
Getting Ready for Change: mental health act amendments for children and young people.	Mental Health Today	Paper
Developments in CAMHS Tier 4 Community-based Service Provision (McDougall et al. 2010)	Royal College of Psychiatrists / Department of Health	Podcast

Source: CSIP (2010).

Step 6: decide how to commission services efficiently

It is important to have clear structures in place so that all partners know how the service is being led, how progress will be evaluated and how decisions are made. A clear plan is needed, but this should be adaptable if the evaluation identifies a need for change. How the project will be contracted should be agreed within this step.

Step 7: commission – including use of pooled resources

Following the preparation and development of a service specification contracting can proceed. This may include recommissioning with a current provider ensuring delivery of effective services with specified outcomes. Alternatively, if commissioning a new provider, requesting tenders, shortlisting, interviewing and contracting will be required. Before starting the process it is helpful to review what outcomes are required, to make sure that both commissioners and the provider are clear from the outset. It is also important to consider what resources are available from other services, both within health and from the local authority, which can be used to support Tier 4 provision.

Step 8: plan for workforce and market development

Commissioning of Tier 4 services will have an impact on the workforce and market across CAMHS. New developments and opportunities will attract staff, so consideration needs to be given as to how to retain staff within the other tiers. Working closely with the workforce deanery to attract staff into CAMHS is one solution. Developments such as the CAMHS Foundation degree offer an entry into CAMHS for non-clinical staff. Developing new roles such as liaison staff can encourage staff to develop within their existing roles.

Step 9: monitor and review services and process

Commissioners need to plan for short-, medium- and long-term monitoring. Criteria for outcomes should be agreed in advance as set out in steps 1 and 5. In the short term this may include verbal feedback such as user feedback or general comments from staff on the new services. More medium-term evaluation of young peoples' views and staff attitudes can be undertaken, as well as an evaluation of clinical outcomes for young people. Long term, at least a year later, the impact on appropriate referral rates, reduction in waiting times and continued improvement in clients clinical outcomes can be measured which will inform the direction of travel for the future.

Completing the cycle

There is a need to use the evaluation systematically to help refine services to ensure they continue to fit the need. Undertaking a needs assessment at a set period can identify where services can be refined and offer opportunities to respond swiftly as new developments, policy and thinking emerge. The cycle can then be implemented again to ensure effective joint commissioning continues.

Summary of The Joint Planning and Commissioning Cycle

The Joint Planning and Commissioning Cycle offers commissioners a stepped approach that can be applied to many services including Tier 4 services. It encourages broad thinking across partners and allows for the development of complex services through needs assessment and service planning. The outcomes of children and young people are at the core, from step 1 to step 9 and around again, ensuring that the focus remains on the needs of the client not the services. Many practical tools have been developed to support the steps. The steps together with the tools provide a comprehensive framework for Tier 4 commissioners.

Commissioning Tier 4 services – the NHS West Midlands experience

Some of the practical issues faced can be illustrated by examining how one local health economy, West Midlands, took the decision to scope and analyse the commissioning of all Tier 4 inpatient stays for children and young people within this geographical area.

Scoping admissions across the area – what did it show?

The scoping phase (i.e. establishing exactly where all children and young people were placed from the existing 17 PCTs) was the first stage in the development of a regional commissioning framework for children and young people requiring this level of care and treatment.

The locality of the West Midlands consists of several urban conurbations (i.e. Birmingham, Wolverhampton and Walsall) and several rural areas (i.e. Shropshire, Staffordshire, Worcestershire and Herefordshire). The population size is over 5 million people with 1 million living within the Birmingham City Council boundary.

Reflecting on the ad hoc commissioning arrangements described earlier, the West Midlands health economy was keen to explore the commissioning improvements (including value for money) that could be achieved through more robust and challenging commissioning arrangements for children and young people with mental health problems requiring admission to hospital.

It was widely known that individual PCTs had to commission their own independent sector placements when the NHS was at full capacity. Thus two different commissioning frameworks already existed. The PCTs' experience of the NHS capacity in turn was not favourable and often the beds were not managed to full commissioned occupancy. This meant that not only were the PCTs funding the NHS capacity through a regional contract, but they were then having to commission and fund individually any admissions within the independent sector. As admissions were not consistent year on year this could be seen as a huge financial risk for each individual PCT as just one admission to a specialised sector unit could cost £100,000s.

For young people this meant that the quality of care was not consistent. No robust monitoring of treatment was in place and often young people could be placed several hundred miles away from their homes. Reviews of adult mental health and social care placements (Ryan et al. 2004) found that without clear review structures and arrangements in place commissioners continued paying for hospital and residential care even when patients were no longer receiving treatment.

The West Midlands CAMHS interim statement of need published in 2008 (Crofts 2008) stated that there was little qualitative data available from the individual PCTs regarding inpatient activity prior to 2007. Therefore, no suggestion of trends could be drawn as they had no validity. This meant that no strategic planning had ever taken place to inform care for this most vulnerable group of children and young people. This still remains the case for many regions in the country today; however, the establishment of commissioning by the NHS Commissioning Board will ensure much more standardisation.

What are young people telling us?

We know from feedback from various sources that a young person's experience of inpatient treatment is very variable and dependent on a number of factors. There is much evidence which identifies and considers patient experience of Tier 4 services. *Where Next?* (Street and Svanberg 2003) found that of the participants they interviewed:

- 26 per cent found the experience of admission a negative one with 20 per cent of those stating it was frightening;
- 67 per cent stated they would have liked more information about their admission;
- 69 per cent wanted to be closer to home;
- Only just over a third – 34 per cent – stated staff were helpful;
- 39 per cent wanted more time with staff; and
- 37 per cent wanted staff to approach them.

The Office of the Children's Commissioner report, *Pushed into the Shadows* (Street 2007), revealed that some young people under 18 do not find it helpful to be admitted to adult psychiatric wards and that it can actually be traumatising and very distressing with no clinical or therapeutic benefit. The resultant changes to the Mental Health Act 1983 regarding the 'age appropriate' environment for under 18s was to help ensure this would not continue.

The national charity 'beat' was commissioned to undertake a user engagement project within the West Midlands CAMHS Tier 4 (beat 2010). They interviewed a number of young people and the four main providers of Tier 4 provision for West Midlands children. Comments around the physical environment were highlighted. These included:

- 'Try making it a warm and welcoming atmosphere and some talk to us as if we're stupid so it needs to improve.'
- 'For it to be individualised rather than generalised.'
- 'Comfier beds.'

The formal peer review process through the Quality Network for Inpatient CAMHS (QNIC), which over 80 per cent of Tier 4 units are members of, also ensures that patient and family experience feature in all reviews.

Regional commissioning – the benefits

Regional or specialised commissioning was, in part, established for high cost and low volume pathways – to develop expertise in commissioning for specific and rare disorders and to make the best use of funding available. If each individual health economy had to pay for treatment for these disorders, when the need arose, this could have a serious and significant financial effect on that commissioning body (formerly the PCTs and latterly the COGS). By collectively bringing commissioning together through a regional collaborative this meant that, first, expertise and knowledge would be gathered by those commissioning on behalf of the collaborative and, second, the risk of serious unplanned financial damage to the individual organisations could be avoided whilst in some cases significant cost savings could potentially be made.

The commissioning landscape is changing again and there will no longer be the regional commissioning groups that existed in 2007. However, the move in the West Midlands to commission all inpatient activity for children and young people with mental health problems by the regional specialised commissioning team was a gallant step which ensured robust performance monitoring was in place at both an individual patient level, i.e. the care and treatment that was directly provided, and at an organisational level. In addition, data and information relating to all inpatient activity could be used therefore to inform a strategy for planning for these young people for the future.

The spend on all Tier 4 inpatient activity at the time the scoping was completed, when calculated as a total for all PCTs, was a phenomenal £17 million. The majority of this was being spent in the independent sector at a high cost for each individual placement.

The model adopted by the West Midlands was one which existed in the regional commissioning of adult mental health secure care. This saw the development of a robust care pathway for all young people requiring inpatient Tier 4 admission driven by and monitored in partnership by the identified commissioner and clinician employed directly by the commissioning team. This ensured a number of key benefits for commissioners of the West Midlands:

- every young person received the most appropriate clinical placement in the best suited environment, based on their needs;
- an open and transparent picture of all providers of each level of care;
- development of 'one' care pathway or journey based on clinical need;
- care and treatment commissioned for each specific disorder/illness based on best evidence, including NICE guidance and effective outcomes;
- comparison of costs and development of a value for money framework;
- individualised care plans initiated for each young person *before* the admission took place;
- robust performance monitoring of each provider;
- each young person placed as close to home as possible;
- collective purchasing power to enable set prices to be established with the independent sector providers and NHS providers.

By developing the pathway described above the West Midlands could begin to strategically plan the future direction to improve services for children and young people who need this level of care. Whereas individual PCTs previously could not plan for these services owing to low numbers, the regional commissioning model ensured that information and data relating to all the West Midlands' children and young people could be used much more effectively to plan provision. This enables identification of a changing demand profile which subsequently can be commissioned for in a systematic way.

The establishment of such a model of care with the above principles was predicated on the involvement of CAMHS clinicians across the region, particularly the local Tier 3 consultant psychiatrists who were keen not to develop a system which was bureaucratic and not user and clinician friendly. A steering group was established and well attended by clinical staff and from that the care pathway was developed. In addition the project lead was a mental health clinician which ensured the eventual process was grounded in clinical terms.

By ensuring clinical and user engagement at all levels and a clear understanding of the rationale for change set out from the beginning, the development of the framework and protocol was seen as achievable and an improvement to existing practice. It can be demonstrated through a partnership approach that much value can be added when commissioning this level of care in this robust way, not least an improved patient journey and standardised performance monitoring across all providers. However, these arrangements do also need to be flexible enough to allow for innovative developments within local areas and not stifle creativity.

In summary, when commissioning services for such a vulnerable group we need to ensure that any service puts the user and their family at the heart of service delivery, with outcomes, both in terms of patient experience and efficacy of treatment, as equally important. In addition, by involving clinicians in the change process and having a clear case for change which identifies key indicators of improvement for young people, the result can be a much more robust and effective pathway. This example demonstrates that a high degree of governance can be obtained even when commissioning a complex service over many providers and for a disparate group of children and young people.

With the inception of NHS England and the development of clinically driven national service specifications for Tier 4, we can anticipate that the commissioning of such complex services will result in more consistent, evidence-based care and treatment for this vulnerable group of children and young people. This model and approach will certainly build upon the achievements within the West Midlands.

West Midlands Specialised Commissioning Group Consultation with Young People

A leading national charity for people affected by eating disorders, beat, were asked by the West Midlands Strategic Commissioning Group to speak to the young people about their treatment and care and their CAMHS Tier 4 strategy. Staff from beat and a beat young ambassador, a person who is in recovery from an eating disorder, spoke to young people of all different ages about:

1   Intensive home treatment – would you like to be treated at home and how often?
2   How can we get more people, from different religions and backgrounds, accessing CAMHS?
3   What does the 'perfect' CAMHS service look like to you?

Eighty-two per cent of the group said that they did not have to wait for inpatient care; however, they said they did have to wait for support and treatment in the early stage of their illness developing. Fifty per cent said they would have preferred to have more treatment at home/closer to home.

Future commissioning arrangements

In 2010 the government set out the future arrangements for commissioning NHS services in England. Local commissioning of secondary care will be undertaken by Clinical Commissioning Groups (CCGs) and NHS England took over the commissioning of national and regional specialised services (Department of Health 2010) from April 2013. These services are defined by:

- number of individuals requiring the provision of the service or facility (rarity);
- the cost of providing the service or facility (infrastructure of specialist centres);
- number of persons able to provide the service or facility (clinical expertise);
- financial implications for CCGs if they were required to arrange for the provision of the service or facility (financial risks).

The list of prescribed specialist services to be commissioned by NHS England is set out in the *Clinical Advisory Group Report* (Department of Health 2012a) and includes Tier 4 CAMHS.

Clinical Reference Groups have been set up for all prescribed services with the task of developing a service specification which can be used nationally. The service specification started to guide specialist commissioners from April 2013, but the Clinical Reference Groups will continue their work to refine and develop the service specification for the future. Specialised commissioning teams within ten nominated Local Area Teams (LATs) commission services within their locality on behalf of NHS England. The LATs use a single operating model for commissioning all prescribed services, introducing an element of uniformity across the country. However, it is intended that any changes in services resulting from the service specification will be introduced gradually to allow time for this to take place. Funding for prescribed services is through a budget determined by NHS England, not via subscriptions or 'top slicing' from the CCGs.

The new model for nationally prescribed services will require consistent pricing, currencies and contracting arrangements. In order to avoid destabilising services in transition a financial envelope will be set with each provider-based on historic levels, but the aim will be to rebase currencies and prices on a national basis for the 2014/15 contracting round. Unlike many services where currencies such as payment by results are well embedded into the commissioning process, it is not clear what currency or currencies will be used for Tier 4 CAMHS.

Even though CAMHS Tier 4 services are commissioned by the LATs, the CCGs will need to understand these specialised services when commissioning local services to ensure that children and young people move across the pathway in a seamless manner. This can be seen as an opportunity to engage in discussions with GPs, looking at the whole range of services and raising the awareness and profile of CAMHS. There will, however, be a large range of competing demands for the CCGs and the challenge for CAMHS commissioners and providers is to raise the mental and emotional health and well-being of young people within their list of priorities.

The local HWBs also play a role in ensuring services are commissioned across a pathway that is from community services right through to complex specialised Tier 4 services. They have statutory responsibilities and bring together the key partners in each area including the local authority, CCGs, NHS England, Local Area Teams, public health and social care. The Director for Children Services is a member of the board. The boards are responsible for supporting joint commissioning and ensuring partnership working within children services. The boards have a key role in ensuring local services meet local needs based on the Joint Strategic Needs Assessment (JSNA) and are able to challenge proposed service provision. That commissioners work with the HWB is important in enabling an integrated approach to CAMHS that meets the needs of health as well as social care and education.

During this time of change in England commissioners will need to work across the new systems. NHS England will have a pivotal role, but CCGs will also play a part and utilising the local HWBs is also important in ensuring an integrated approach.

Summary

Strategic commissioning of any service should be based on good quality and evidence-based assessment of need. Specialist CAMHS and particularly Tier 4 provision have traditionally not been commissioned based on need but through historical and local idiosyncrasies. High quality integrated commissioning is a complex process. Many children and young people experiencing mental health difficulties requiring what are defined in this book as hospital, intensive community and home-based services will undoubtedly come into contact with several agencies such as social care, education support services and healthcare. These agencies commission services in various ways which are then provided differently. Navigating this process requires strong leadership from commissioners who have good relationships with their clinical colleagues.

References

Audit Commission. (2003) *Making Ends Meet*. London: HMSO.
beat. (2010) *Consultation into Tier 4 Services*. Birmingham: West Midlands Specialised Commissioning. Team.
Cotgrove, A., McLoughlin, R., O'Herlihy, A. & Lelliott, P. (2007) The ability of adolescent units to accept emergency admissions: changes in England and Wales between 2000 and 2005. *Psychiatric Bulletin*, 31(12): 457–459.
Crofts, M. (2008) *Interim Statement of Need – CAMHS Tier 4* Birmingham: West Midlands Specialised Commissioning Team.

Department for Education and Skills. (2006) *The Joint Planning and Commissioning Cycle.* London: HMSO.

Department of Health. (2012) *Securing Equity and Excellence in Commissioning Specialised Services.* HMSO, London.

Department of Health. (2012a) *Clinical Advisory Group Report.* London: HMSO.

Department of Health. (2012b) *Prescribed Services: Commissioning Intentions for 2013/14.* London: HMSO.

Hipkiss, H. (2011) *Patient Stories, Visit to Darwin Centre.*

Knapp, M., McDaid, D. & Parsonage, M. (2011) *Mental Health Promotion And Mental Illness Prevention: The economic case.* London: Department of Health.

Kurtz, Z. (2007) *Regional Review of Tier 4 Child and Adolescent Mental Health Services.* London: Department of Health.

National CAMHS Support Service. (2011) *Better Mental Health Outcomes for Children and Young People: A resource directory for commissioners.* London: Department of Health.

O'Herlihy, A., Lelliott, P., Bannister, D., Cotgrove, A., Farr, H. & Tullock, S. (2007) Provision of child and adolescent mental health inpatient services in England between 1999 and 2006. *Psychiatric Bulletin,* 31(12): 454–456.

Royal College of Psychiatrists. (2006) *Building and Sustaining Specialist Child and Adolescent Mental Health Services.* London: RCP.

Rutter, M. (1987) Resilience in the face of adversity: protective factors and resistance to psychiatric disorder. *British Journal of Psychiatry,* 147: 598–611.

Ryan, T., Pearsall, A., Hatfield, B. & Poole, R. (2004) A pilot study of out of area placements for serious mental illness in the private sector. *Journal of Mental Health,* 13(4): 425–429.

Street, C. (2007) *Pushed into the Shadows – Young People's Experience of Adult Mental Health Services.* London: Office of the Children's Commissioner.

Street, C. & Svanberg, J. (2003) *Where Next? New directions in in-patient mental health services for young people. Report 2. Issues emerging: views from young people, parents and staff.* London: YoungMinds.

West Midlands Specialised Commissioning Team. (2009). *CAMHS Tier 4 Strategy and Implementation Plan 2009–2014.* Birmingham: WMSCT.

Worrell, A. et al. (2004) Inappropriate admission of young people with mental disorder to adult psychiatric wards and paediatric wards: cross sectional study of six months' activity. *British Medical Journal,* 328(7444): 867.

13

QUALITY STANDARDS FOR SPECIALIST MENTAL HEALTHCARE SERVICES

Tim McDougall and Peter Thompson

Key points

- Quality standards assist service providers to demonstrate that they are providing care and treatment of a high calibre and to benchmark themselves against similar organisations.
- Membership of a quality network and service accreditation can be used to demonstrate the quality of a service to young people, parents, commissioners and referrers.
- The large majority of inpatient units in the UK are members of the Quality Network for Inpatient CAMHS (QNIC) which has set standards for quality, safety and patient involvement in inpatient units. The Quality Network for Community CAMHS provides a similar framework for community services.
- Standards for safe and appropriate care for young people on adult mental health wards have been developed to support mental health commissioners and providers to meet their obligations under the Mental Health Act 1983. The amendments to the Act enable young people to be admitted to adult wards if their needs are 'atypical' or 'overriding'.
- As part of guideline implementation, the National Institute for Health and Care Excellence (NICE) have started to publish quality standards as benchmarks of high quality and cost-effective patient care. These are likely to have a growing influence on the delivery of inpatient care in the future.

Introduction

Clinical and quality standards are increasingly part of the governance of hospital, intensive community and home-based services.

The National Quality Board recommends that mental health provider organisations use nationally recognised quality standards and produce quality accounts to benchmark their performance (Department of Health 2011a).

No Health without Mental Health, the government's mental health outcomes strategy (Department of Health 2011b), takes a life course approach and includes guidance on improving inpatient services. Among other things, it calls for quality standards to improve the safety and effectiveness of inpatient services.

Which standards apply to CAMHS?

A range of quality standards apply to hospital, community and home-based services, and these provide a way of benchmarking and evaluating services (McDougall et al. 2008). Some standards are essential, others are highly recommended and a few are optional.

Care Quality Commission essential standards of quality and safety

The Care Quality Commission (CQC) in England is the independent regulatory body responsible for reviewing and inspecting the quality of care provided in all hospitals, care homes and care services. The CQC now plays a key role in ensuring NHS trusts and independent sector providers comply with the 'age-appropriate' amendments to the Mental Health Act 1983 (Gillen 2010). The current CQC essential standards have been developed to regulate a wide range of settings, including children and young people in a psychiatric inpatient setting.

Inpatient CAMHS

Inpatient services for vulnerable people have been very much in the public focus over the last few years. The safety of our services, the quality of interventions we provide and how well we engage young people have each been priorities.

In mental health there has not been a consistent set of definitions that describes what is meant by an inpatient bed. This has led to difficulty in benchmarking and understanding patterns of performance (Mental Health Network NHS Confederation 2012). The National Inpatient Child and Adolescent Psychiatry Study (NICAPS; O'Herlihy et al. 1999) developed and piloted a set of service standards based on the available evidence, national policy, best practice guidance and the views of stakeholders. NICAPS noted significant variance in practice and, as a result, the Quality Network for Inpatient CAMHS (QNIC) was launched in 2001 to review inpatient CAMHS units against a set of comprehensive service standards. The standards include environment and facilities; staffing and training; care and treatment; information, consent and confidentiality; and rights and safeguards.

Starting with 36 units over a decade ago the network now comprises over 100 inpatient units which is over 90 per cent of all inpatient units in the UK. There are also units in the Republic of Ireland, Iceland, Norway and Turkey, which are members. At the end of cycle 11, most were achieving high standards in all seven areas of quality that the process focuses on (see Figure 13.1).

Participating services score themselves against the QNIC standards in a self-review. They then receive a peer review when a team of clinicians from other services around the UK visit the service to help them reflect on their self-review and to develop action plans

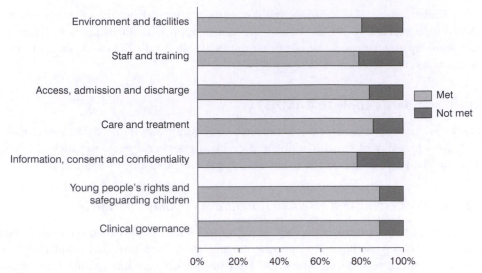

FIGURE 13.1 QNIC essential standards (Royal College of Psychiatrists 2012b)

to meet any unmet standards. As part of the review day, the review team meet with staff, young people and parents/carers.

After each peer or accreditation review, the QNIC team produce individual service reports. Each year an annual report is published which aggregates the data from all members to identify key themes facing inpatient services. This provides important information about the quality of services, which appear to be improving each year (Royal College of Psychiatrists 2012b). QNIC also compare the data collected year on year to identify where improvements have occurred. For example, in 2005 only 55 per cent of staff were receiving clinical supervision, whereas this was 76 per cent in 2011. With such a large number of services participating in QNIC, this provides a regularly updated data set showing trends in inpatient CAMHS services throughout the country.

QNIC have also shared the aggregated data with the Department of Health and previously with the National Advisory Council for Children's Mental Health and Psychological Wellbeing and the National CAMHS Support Service to support the need for ongoing strategic development within CAMHS.

In 2011 QNIC developed the option of accreditation by the Royal College of Psychiatrists. This is a more robust process requiring more self-review data to be collected and for evidence to be shown on the peer review day. Four levels of accreditation are available:

1   accredited as excellent;
2   accredited;
3   deferred;
4   not accredited.

QNIC has been able to assist members in the quality assurance process by providing support in such areas as the collection of outcome measurement data and service user involvement. There is an annual conference where members are encouraged to share innovative practice and also special interest days are held which look at topics in-depth which many services are finding challenging. Past topics have included consent and capacity and education in inpatient CAMHS.

In 2010 QNIC also started to recruit young people advisors. They represent the opinions of young people at all stages of the QNIC process including during the development of standards and as part of review teams visiting inpatient services.

QNIC Routine Outcome Measurement

Service providers are urged to measure outcomes as part of the implementation of the *National Service Framework for Children, Young People and Maternity Services* (Department of Health 2004). Since 2007 QNIC member units have had the option of joining QNIC Routine Outcome Measurement (ROM) Service, which is a collaborative project with the CAMHS Outcomes Research Consortium (CORC). This allows inpatient units to compare their data and inform priorities for service development and evaluation (CAMHS Outcomes Research Consortium 2007). QNIC ROM comprises the following outcome measures including some optional measures such as the CAMHS Service Satisfaction Scale (CAMHSSS; Ayton et al. 2007) (see Box 13.1).

Young people on adult mental health wards

The *National Service Framework for Children, Young People and Maternity Services* set the expectation that young people admitted to hospital for mental health treatment should have access to appropriate care in an environment suited to their age and development (Department of Health 2004). An age appropriate environment refers not just to physical accommodation, but also to the staff and facilities that children and young people need to fulfil their personal, social and educational development whilst in hospital.

Section 31 of the Mental Health Act 2007 amends the Mental Health Act 1983 to place a duty on hospital managers to ensure that patients under 18 admitted to hospital for mental disorder are accommodated in an environment that is suitable for their age (subject to their needs). This is set out in section 131A of the Mental Health Act 1983 and the provision applies to both informal and detained patients. Following what became known as the 'age appropriate environment' amendment the National Institute for Mental Health in England (NIMHE) and the Royal College of Psychiatrists Centre for Quality

---

BOX 13.1   QNIC Routine Outcome Measurement Service

1   Health of the Nation Outcome Scales (Child and Adolescent Mental Health) (HoNOSCA) (self-rated/parent rated) (Gowers et al. 1999).
2   Children's Global Assessment Scale (CGAS) of Functioning (Shaffer et al. 1983).
3   Strengths and Difficulties Questionnaire (SDQ) (Goodman 1997).

TABLE 13.1 Safe and Appropriate Care for Young People on Adult Mental Health Wards: overriding and atypical needs

Overriding	Atypical
When a young person needs immediate admission for their safety or that of others. This acknowledges that, although an inpatient adolescent bed is normally the preferred environment, there will be occasions when an adolescent bed (or alternative such as intensive outreach / crisis service) is not available. The revised Code of Practice (2008) states that if a young person is admitted in a crisis it should be for the briefest time possible (see 36.71).	When, even if an adolescent bed was available, an adult mental health ward is the most appropriate environment. For example, a young person who is nearly 18, who has left school and is being treated by the Early Intervention Psychosis team may be appropriately admitted. However, even in these circumstances or where a young person chooses to be treated in an adult ward as an alternative to an adolescent unit, safeguards must be in place to protect their welfare.

Source: O'Herlihy et al. (2009).

Improvement (CCQI) jointly published standards for safe and appropriate care for young people on adult mental health wards (O'Herlihy et al. 2009). This was partly to help address some of the confusion about what constituted a safe and appropriate environment for young people (Pugh 2008).

For all children under 16 and most young people aged 16 or 17 who require an inpatient mental health service, the most appropriate environment will be a child or adolescent inpatient unit. However, young people aged 16 or 17 can be admitted to adult mental health wards if this is the most suitable environment to meet their needs. In the exceptional case where a young person cannot be accommodated in a CAMHS unit, discrete accommodation within an adult mental health ward is permissible if there is support from CAMHS staff, robust safeguarding measures and age appropriate facilities are available. In determining whether the environment is suitable, hospital managers are required to consult a person whom they consider to be suitable because of their experience in child and adolescent mental health.

The standards for *Safe and Appropriate Care for Young People on Adult Mental Health Wards* (O'Herlihy et al. 2009) refer to young people with 'overriding' or 'atypical' needs (see Table 13.1).

The standards for *Safe and Appropriate Care for Young People on Adult Mental Health Wards* are a 'toolkit' designed to help adult mental health service providers assess how well they are meeting the needs of young people aged under 18. Some statements reflect statutory requirements and others are consensus statements derived from best practice. Consequently, not all adult mental health wards are expected to meet every criterion.

The criteria for safe and appropriate care on adult mental health wards were adapted from the Adult Inpatient Mental Health Services (AIMS) standards and the QNIC. For wards using the AIMS standards, the *Safe and Appropriate Care for Young People on Adult Mental Health Wards* are intended to be complementary. The criteria are either rated as essential, expected or desirable and have been organised into seven sections (see Tables 13.2 and 13.3).

TABLE 13.2 Safe and Appropriate Care for Young People on Adult Mental Health Wards: rating scheme

Code	Rating	Definition
1	Essential	Failure to meet these criteria would result in a significant threat to patient safety, rights or dignity and would breach the law.
2	Expected	Criteria that would indicate good practice and that a ward should be expected to meet.
3	Desirable	Criteria that an excellent ward should meet or criteria that are not the direct responsibility of the ward.

Source: Adapted from the AIMS standards (O'Herlihy et al 2009).

TABLE 13.3 Safe and Appropriate Care for Young People on Adult Mental Health Wards: key standards

Section 1	Environment and facilities
	These criteria focus on the ward's physical accommodation and the availability of facilities suitable for young people.
Section 2	Staffing and training
	These criteria focus on the general staffing and training needs of wards that are preparing to provide safe and appropriate care for young people.
Section 3	Assessment, admission, transfers and discharge
	These criteria focus on procedures for admission, transfers and discharge.
Section 4	Care and treatment
	These criteria outline the staff and services required to plan the care of young people admitted, care planning, and the activities young people should expect to have access to during their admission, no matter how brief their stay.
Section 5	Education and further learning
	These criteria apply to young people admitted with an atypical need, whose expected stay on an adult mental health ward may be longer than a few days.
Section 6	Information, consent, confidentiality and advocacy
	These criteria outline the information young people and parents or carers can expect to receive, their right to age appropriate advocacy, and the procedures and processes that should be followed when obtaining consent and managing confidentiality.
Section 7	Other safeguards
	This section outlines additional safeguards that must be considered when young people are placed on adult mental health wards, no matter how brief their stay.

Quality Network for Community CAMHS

Formerly known as the Quality Network for Multi agency CAMHS (QINMAC), the Quality Network for Community Child and Adolescent Mental Health Services (QNCC) was established by the Royal College of Psychiatrists Centre for Quality Improvement in 2005 and the inaugural standards were published in 2006. The QNCC standards are now in their third edition (Royal College of Psychiatrists 2012b).

QNCC has developed a set of standards for generic and learning disability CAMHS services, as well as a subset for services which provide a crisis and/or intensive interventions. The subset has been developed through a review of policy and strategy and good practice guidance, and is based on service protocols from several intensive community and home-based services for children and young people CAMHS teams in the UK. The subset should be read alongside the main standards (see Table 13.4).

The standards follow a care pathway, and emphasise multi-agency working. They address aspects of policy including the CQC's *Essential Standards of Quality and Safety* (CQC 2010), the Welsh Assembly Government's *Healthcare Standards for Wales* (Welsh Assembly Government 2010) and Scotland's *Delivering a Healthy Future* (Scottish Executive 2007). Services across the UK can therefore use their review reports to demonstrate compliance with these national standards.

TABLE 13.4 QNCC crisis and/or intensive response subset

Defining theme	Description
Immediate response	Able to respond to requests for immediate CAMHS support, within a few hours of receiving the request.
'Out-of-hours' availability (including on-call rota)	CAMHS response available 24 hours/7 days a week or with 'out-of-hours' cover and access to a professional who can undertake a Mental Health Act assessment at any hour required.
Assertive approach to engagement	Persistent approach to engagement – repeated attempts at contact (e.g. follow up non-attendance directly with young people by phone/text, flexible about meeting another time, etc.).
Flexible contact arrangements	Working with young people in locations that are safe but where they are happy to meet and engage, and at a time that suits them. Contacts may vary from face to face or phone meetings, or home or school visits.
Planned intensive intervention and support in the community	Intensive clinical input involving three to five contacts a week, and high staff to service user ratio until the need for intensive input is resolved.
Support the stepped care approach for those in need	Able to provide continuity of managed care to standard community, day- or inpatient CAMHS care as required.
Collaborative working relationships with, other multidisciplinary CAMHS professionals, local services and agencies	Able to access other CAMHS professionals, and/or agencies as required in order to meet the needs of the young person and their parents/carers.

Like its sister service QNIC, QNCC is a peer review network which includes a self-review. Self-review membership means that services are not visited by other CAMHS teams, but they do get a report which can help benchmark the quality of their services. Some provider trusts which provide several discrete CAMHS teams alternate between self and peer review membership to enable them to keep all their teams signed up within a limited budget.

Services that have participated in at least one cycle of review are eligible to apply for accreditation. This enables providers to demonstrate the quality of care and treatment they offer to children and young people, parents and carers and service commissioners. Accreditation is awarded by the Royal College of Psychiatrists and lasts for three years.

Quality Network for Eating Disorders

The CCQI also have a Quality Network for Eating Disorders (QED). The QED standards are specific to providing eating disorder care and are intended to be read alongside the QNIC and QNCC standards for CAMHS and the AIMS standards for adult inpatient services.

The Royal College of Psychiatrists have also developed guidance on the management of children and young people with anorexia nervosa (Royal College of Psychiatrists 2012c; Junior MARSIPAN). This has been endorsed by professional organisations, eating disorders charities, and children and young people themselves.

The guidelines build on a report from the joint Royal College of Psychiatrists & Royal College of Physicians (2010) Management of Really Sick Patients with Anorexia Nervosa (MARSIPAN) group. The Junior report covers various aspects of care and treatment for children and young people with anorexia nervosa (see Box 13.2).

BOX 13.2   Junior MARSIPAN

- risk assessment, physical examination and associated action;
- location of care and transition between services;
- compulsory treatment;
- paediatric admission and local protocols;
- management of re-feeding;
- management of compensatory behaviours associated with an eating disorder in a paediatric setting;
- management in primary care and paediatric out-patient settings;
- discharge from paediatric settings;
- management in specialist CAMHS in-patient settings.

Source: Royal College of Psychiatrists (2012c).

Other quality standards

In addition to the standards published by the Royal College of Psychiatrists there are a number of other quality criteria and guidelines. These include the Department of Health's (2007) *You're Welcome* standards and the Health and Social Care Advisory Service's (2008) participation standards. The National Institute for Health and Care Excellence are also starting to publish quality standards as part of their range of NICE guidelines.

You're Welcome

The *You're Welcome* quality criteria (Department of Health 2007) set standards for NHS and independent providers of health services to be 'young people friendly' including a section on targeted and specialist CAMHS (see Box 13.3).

The *You're Welcome* standards are self-assessed but the process includes external verification and moderation. The self-assessment process is designed to enable services to work towards achieving a formal '*You're Welcome*' quality benchmark. It is the government vision that the majority of settings providing healthcare for young people will achieve the *You're Welcome* status by 2020.

Young people's participation

The Health and Social Care Advisory Service has published standards focusing on young people's participation (Health and Social Care Advisory Service 2008). Rather than exploring the views of individual children and young people, the standards take a systemic approach to address service organisation, organisational structures and the wider partnership context. Included as part of the implementation toolkit was a self-assessment to support health service providers ensure that children and young people's views are systematically sought and incorporated into reviews of service provision.

Substance misuse

The Royal College of General Practitioners and CCQI have collaborated with DrugScope and Alcohol Concern to produce practice standards for young people with substance misuse problems (Royal College of Psychiatrists 2012a). These are linked to the QNCC standards and focus on:

- identification and brief assessment;
- comprehensive assessment;
- integrated care planning;
- integrated care and interventions;
- planned completion and transfer of care.

The standards are based on NICE guidance, systematic reviews and national substance misuse policies and strategies. They emphasise a sensitive, non-judgemental and collaborative

BOX 13.3 *You're Welcome* Quality Criteria: specialist child and adolescent mental health services and facilities that offer specialist services

The service provides young people, their parents and carers with:
- advice and information to help informed decision making;
- information materials to help informed decision making;
- information and advice explaining the roles of staff they might encounter in mental health services.

All appropriate staff routinely discuss choices with young people:
- young people and their families are offered information and advice to facilitate informed decision making;
- discussions take place at the beginning and throughout therapeutic contact.

The services offer information and advice to help young people and their families to make decisions regarding their psychological wellbeing and mental health support needs, and treatment choices based on informed consent. The service makes routine attempts to provide flexibility about involving other people in the assessment and treatment process.

Appropriate staff receive training and appraisal to ensure that they are:
- able to talk to young people about mental health issues;
- knowledgeable about a range of support and treatment options;
- clear about what they can and cannot do to help young people;
- clear about who they are able to help;
- able to recognise and respond to different therapeutic needs such as those relating to gender, gender identity, sexual orientation, ethnicity and age, disability, religion or belief;
- able to recognise and facilitate informed consent.

Services are flexible about involving other people in the assessment and treatment process, particularly at first contact, and:

Young people are offered appropriate information and advice to help them understand what can be achieved without parental or family involvement wherever this is considered to be therapeutically beneficial. Refusal of consent to family involvement is accepted unless there is serious risk to the young person's welfare

Even when assertive action is needed, there is some flexibility about what choices can be made available and which treatment the young person would like to receive. Even in cases where the overriding serious risks lead to compulsory treatment, young people should always be offered appropriate information and advice to make treatment choices based on informed consent.

Source: Department of Health (2007)

BOX 13.4   Practice standards for young people with substance misuse problems

Essential

These are minimum standards and criteria that are critical to care. Failure to meet these standards and criteria would result in a significant threat to patient safety, rights or dignity and/or would breach the law.

Expected

These are standards and criteria that a professional and/or team providing a good service would be expected to meet, and that young people and parents and carers should expect to receive.

Desirable

Criteria that indicate excellent practice and care. They may not be the direct responsibility of staff, professionals or services.

---

approach to supporting children and young people with substance misuse problems. Like other standards produced by the CCQI the criteria and standards that underpin them are rated as essential, desirable and expected (see Box 13.4).

NICE quality standards

There is a growing range of clinical guidelines that include children and young people in their scope, and most major mental health and developmental disorders are now covered. Some guidelines have included standards-based interactive clinical pathways as part of the wider guideline. For example, the depression in children guideline includes information on transfer from CAMHS to adult services (National Collaborating Centre for Mental Health 2005)

The Health and Social Care Act 2012 sets out a new responsibility for NICE to develop quality standards and other guidance for social care in England. As part of clinical guideline implementation, NICE have started to publish quality standards as benchmarks of high quality and cost-effective patient care. These focus on clinical effectiveness, patient safety and patient experience and are likely to have a growing influence on the delivery of inpatient care in the future. This is likely to be through incentive schemes such as the Commissioning for Quality and Innovation (CQUIN) and Quality and Outcomes Framework (QOF) frameworks. A number of clinical standards that focus on children and young people are currently in development. These include those focused on depression in children and young people; attention deficit hyperactivity disorder (ADHD); and the health and well-being of looked after children.

Summary

Quality standards provide clinicians, commissioners and users of hospital, intensive community and home-based services with benchmarks with which they can measure performance and the standard of care. They are sourced from the best available evidence as well as the consensus views of clinical experts. The CCQI have led the way in setting quality standards that apply to hospital, intensive community and home-based services. These offer providers a framework within which they can continuously improve the care and treatment they give to children and young people.

References

Ayton, A., Mooney, M., Sillifant, K., Powls, J. & Rasool, H. (2007). The development of the child and adolescent versions of the Verona Service Satisfaction Scale (CAMHSSS). *Social Psychiatry and Psychiatric Epidemiology*, 42(11), 892–901.

CAMHS Outcomes Research Consortium. (2007). www.corc.uk.net/index.php

Care Quality Commission. (2010). *Essential Standards of Quality and Safety*. London: CQC.

Department of Health. (2004). *National Service Framework for Children, Young People and Maternity Services*. London: HMSO.

Department of Health. (2007). *You're Welcome Quality Criteria: making health services young people friendly*. London: HMSO.

Department of Health. (2011a). *Quality Governance in the NHS: a guide for provider boards*. London: HMSO.

Department of Health. (2011b). *No Health without Mental Health: a cross government mental health outcomes strategy for people of all ages*. London: HMSO.

Gillen, S. (2010). The dying art. professional social work, September, 20–21.

Goodman, R. (1997). The Strengths and Difficulties Questionnaire: a research note. *Journal of Child Psychology and Psychiatry*, 38, 581–586.

Gowers, S. G., Harrington, R. C., Whitton, A., et al. (1999) Brief scale for measuring the outcomes of emotional and behavioural disorders in children: Health of the Nation Outcome Scales for Children and Adolescents (HoNOSCA). *British Journal of Psychiatry*, 174, 413–416.

Health and Social Care Advisory Service. (2008). *Quality Standards for Children and Young People's Participation in CAMHS*. London: HASCAS.

McDougall, T., Worrall-Davies, A., Hewson, L., Richardson, G. & Cotgrove, A. (2008). Tier 4 Child and Adolescent Mental Health Services: inpatient care, day services and alternatives: an overview of Tier 4 CAMHS provision in the UK. *Child and Adolescent Mental Health*, 13(4) 173–180.

Mental Health Network NHS Confederation. (2012). *Defining Mental Health Services: promoting effective commissioning and supporting QIPP*. London: MHNNC.

National Collaborating Centre for Mental Health. (2005). *Depression in Children and Young People: identification and management in primary, community and secondary care. National Clinical Practice Guideline Number 28*. London. NICE.

O'Herlihy, A., Worrall, A., Banerjee S., Jaffa, T., Mears, P., Brook, H., Scott, A., White, R., Nikolaou, V. & Lelliot, P. (1999). *National Inpatient Child and Adolescent Psychiatry Study (NICAPS). Initial report to the Department of Health*. London: Royal College of Psychiatrists Research Unit.

O'Herlihy, A., et al. (2009) *Safe and Appropriate Care for Young People on Adult Mental Health Wards*. The Royal College of Psychiatrists Centre for Quality Improvement. Royal College of Psychiatrists, National Mental Health Development Unit, National Patient Safety Agency.

Pugh, K. (2008). Getting ready for change. *Mental Health Today*, July/August, 29–31.

Royal College of Psychiatrists. (2012a). *Practice Standards for Young People with Substance Misuse Problems.* London: CCQI.

Royal College of Psychiatrists. (2012b).*Quality Network for Inpatient CAMHS: annual report, cycle 12.* London: CCQI.

Royal College of Psychiatrists. (2012c). *Management of Really Sick Patients under 18 with Anorexia Nervosa (College Report CR168).* London: Royal College of Psychiatrists.

Royal College of Psychiatrists & Royal College of Physicians. (2010). *MARSIPAN: Management of Really Sick Patients with Anorexia Nervosa (College Report CR162).* London: Royal College of Psychiatrists.

Scottish Executive. (2007). *Delivering a Health Future: an action framework for children and young people's health in Scotland.* Edinburgh: Scottish Executive.

Shaffer, D., Gould, M. & Brasic, J. (1983). A Children's Global Assessment Scale (CGAS). *Archives of General Psychiatry,* 40, 1228–1231.

Welsh Assembly Government. (2010). *Doing Well, Doing Better: standards for health services in Wales.* Cardiff: WAG.

14

THE LEGAL FRAMEWORK

Camilla Parker

Key points

- All decisions concerning the delivery of mental healthcare to a child or young person, whether relating to treatment or planning or commissioning services, must be undertaken in the context of human rights and equality law. Those working with children and young people will need to identify the person(s) with parental responsibility for them.
- Children and young people receiving care and treatment from Tier 4 CAMHS will have wide-ranging, and often complex, needs. They are likely to need support in addition to the mental healthcare that they are receiving. It is therefore vital that CAMHS professionals work closely with other services within the NHS, and local social services authorities (both children and adult) as well as other relevant agencies, such as housing, to ensure that children and young people receive the support that they need.
- Where inpatient treatment is considered to be the most appropriate means of providing a child or young person with the treatment and care that s/he needs, the legal basis for the admission and treatment must be determined. This is an area in which amendments to the Mental Health Act 1983 (the MHA 1983) by the Mental Health Act 2007 and revisions to the MHA Code have introduced significant changes, such as the age appropriate environment duty (section 131A of the MHA 1983). Mental health professionals will need to be aware of the circumstances in which under 18s can be admitted informally (on the basis of their consent, parental consent or, in relation to 16- and 17-year-olds, by relying on the Mental Capacity Act 2005) and when admission under the MHA 1983 should be considered.
- All children and young people detained under the MHA 1983 should be informed of, and supported in exercising, their rights. This includes being informed about the section of the MHA 1983 under which they are detained, what this means in practice (including the treatment provisions under Part 4 of the Act), and the right to apply to the Mental Health Tribunal. The MHA Code states that informal patients should also be made aware of their rights.

- The MHA 1983 includes provisions for the care and treatment of individuals living in the community, which may be relevant to children and young people receiving mental healthcare from Tier 4 CAMHS, namely section 17 leave, guardianship and supervised community treatment (SCT).

Introduction

This chapter provides an overview of the legal framework relevant to children and young people receiving treatment and support from Tier 4 Child and Adolescent Mental Health Services (CAMHS). Practitioners will be aware that the provision of mental healthcare to children and young people, whether in hospital or in community-based settings, engages a wide range of complex and interrelating legislation and policy. Given that an examination of every relevant aspect is not possible within a single chapter, this chapter focuses on areas likely to be of key importance for CAMHS practitioners in relation to their work, including engaging with other agencies that also have responsibilities for the care and support of children and young people with severe mental health problems. The following four main areas are covered:

1   access to services and support;
2   admission and treatment in hospital;
3   rights in hospital;
4   compulsory powers in the community.

In addition to summarising the key issues for each of these areas, issues lacking legal clarity and/or raising new or difficult questions are considered. Information on where to obtain further information and guidance is provided throughout the text. A list of useful resources is also provided at the end of this chapter.

Terminology

As law and policy differs slightly between these two age groups, those under 16 are referred to as a 'child' or 'children' and those aged 16 or 17 are referred to as a 'young person' or 'young people'. This adopts the terminology used by the Code of Practice to the Mental Health Act (the MHA Code).[1]

Overarching principles and concepts

All decisions concerning the delivery of mental healthcare to a child or young person, whether they are concerned with treatment or planning or commissioning services, must be undertaken in the context of human rights and equality law.[2] The requirement to respect children and young people's right to confidentiality[3] and involve them in the planning and delivery of their care are also core overarching principles for CAMHS, whether provided in the community or in hospital.

Parental responsibility

All those working with children and young people will be aware of the importance of identifying the person(s) with parental responsibility for them.[4] Not only is it good practice to involve those with parental responsibility (subject to the child/young person's consent), but in some circumstances those with parental responsibility will be able to authorise the proposed intervention, such as admission to hospital or treatment for the child or young person's mental health problems. Such consent can only be relied on if the decision falls within the 'zone of parental control' – this is discussed below.

Access to services and support

Children and young people receiving care and treatment from Tier 4 CAMHS will have wide-ranging and often complex needs, reflecting their diverse backgrounds, cultures and experience. For example, some may have physical and/or learning disabilities in addition to severe mental health problems, some may be seeking asylum, some may have been sexually abused, some may have special educational needs, some may be 'looked after children' and some may be involved with the youth justice system.

All these children and young people, but particularly those receiving services in the community, or about to be discharged from inpatient care, are likely to need additional support to the mental healthcare that they are receiving. This may include support to their parents, or other relatives providing informal care. Many young people who are reaching an age when they are too old to continue to receive CAMHS will need support as they make the transition into adult life. For example, in addition to their mental health needs, these young people may require suitable accommodation, further education or training, or practical support in getting a job.

To help children and young people receive the support that they need, it is vital that CAMHS professionals work closely with other services within the NHS, in particular adult mental health services, and local social services authorities (both children and adult) as well as other relevant agencies, such as housing, youth justice and the voluntary sector. The importance of joint working is emphasised in a range of mental health policies, such as *Refocusing the Care Programme Approach*,[5] and underpinned by the duty on NHS bodies and local authorities to cooperate expressed in legislation such as the Children Act 2004 (section 10) and the NHS Act 2006 (section 82).

The legal framework for access to health and social care services is examined in detail in *Transitions in Mental Health Care*.[6] While its focus is on young people making the transition from CAMHS to adult services, *Transitions in Mental Health Care* covers the range of legislation and policy relevant to the assessment of health and social care needs and decisions on the services to be provided to meet such needs for children, young people and adults. It also considers the responsibilities of local authorities to 'looked after children', carers' assessments, direct payments and personal budgets.

One area that may give rise to confusion or uncertainty is the responsibilities of local authorities in relation to children and young people receiving mental healthcare from CAMHS. The definition of a 'child in need' for the purpose of section 17 of the Children

Act 1989 (the CA 1989) is considered below, followed by the scope of the duty to assess under section 47 of the NHS and Community Care Act 1990.

Children in need and the Children Act 1989

While the scope of their duties will differ depending on the age and situation of the individual, it is clear that local authorities should ensure that all such children and young people receive an assessment of their needs. In most cases the assessment will be carried out under section 17 of the CA 1989 which requires local authorities to safeguard and promote the welfare of children 'in need' in their area by providing 'a range and level of services appropriate to those children's needs'. Those children and young people under 18 who are receiving mental healthcare from CAMHS will be considered to be 'a child in need' as this term includes those who 'suffer from a mental disorder of any kind'.

Alternatively (for example, if it is argued that the child or young person has no diagnosis and it is not clear that s/he has a mental disorder) children and young people who have been assessed to need support from CAMHS should be considered to be a 'child in need' because their '...health or development is likely to be significantly impaired, or further impaired', without the provision of such services.[7]

Section 17 CA 1989 assessments may also incorporate an assessment under section 2 of the Chronically Sick and Disabled Person Act 1970 which places a duty on social services to provide certain services, such as practical assistance in the home, that they have assessed a disabled person[8] to need.

Community care assessments under the NHS and Community Care Act 1990

Some under 18s may be entitled to an assessment under section 47 of the NHS and Community Care Act 1990, for example because section 117 of the Mental Health Act 1983 applies to them, following their discharge from hospital.[9]

Section 47 requires local authorities to carry out an assessment of the needs of individuals who may be in need of 'community care services' (this term includes a wide range of services such as social work service advice and support, domiciliary care, assistance in finding accommodation and residential care). This duty:

- arises when the social services authority is made aware that a person may be in need of such services;
- applies whether or not the young person is considered to meet the criteria for receiving care from adult mental health services under the Care Programme Approach;
- should be applied to young people who are about to become 18 and are likely to need community services as an adult (they should be treated as a 'person who may be in need' of community care services).[10]

Admission and treatment in hospital

Wherever possible, children and young people should be provided with the support that they need while living at home. This is consistent with human rights principles, such as Article 8 (the right to family and private life) of the European Convention on Human Rights – while an interference of this right may be permitted in certain circumstances, such as for the protection of the person's health, this must be a proportionate response to the concern being addressed. However, there will be circumstances in which a period of inpatient treatment is considered to be the most appropriate means of providing a child or young person with the treatment and care that s/he needs. In such cases, the legal basis for the admission and treatment must be determined.

This is an area in which amendments to the Mental Health Act 1983 (the MHA 1983) by the Mental Health Act 2007 (the MHA 2007) and revisions to the MHA Code have introduced significant changes. For example the age appropriate environment duty under section 131A of the MHA 1983 places a duty on hospital managers to ensure that the hospital environment in which a child or young person is to be accommodated is suitable for that patient, having regard to the patient's age, subject to his or her needs. This duty applies to all patients under 18, whether they are liable to be detained or admitted to hospital as an informal patient (including those who have been admitted informally on the basis of parental consent).[11]

Set out below is a brief overview of the key aspects relating to the admission to hospital and treatment of children and young people, followed by areas identified as meriting further consideration. Further information is provided in *The Legal Aspects of the Care and Treatment of Children and Young People with Mental Disorder: A Guide for Professionals.*[12] In addition, the National Mental Health Development Unit produced two flow charts, designed to assist mental health professionals in ascertaining whether a child or young person can be admitted informally, or whether detention under the MHA 1983 should be considered. One is for young people (*Admission to Hospital and Treatment for Mental Disorder: Young People aged 16 or 17 years old* [13]) and the other is for children (Admission to Hospital and Treatment for Mental Disorder: Children under 16 years old[14]).

Informal admission and/or treatment

Children and young people able to decide

A child or young person who is able to make such decisions can consent or refuse to be admitted to hospital and/or treated for their mental disorder.

Respecting the competent refusal of a child or young person is an important change. In relation to the admission of young people, in addition to providing that they can consent to their admission to hospital, irrespective of their parent's views, section 131 MHA 1983 now prohibits parental consent from overriding a young person's refusal. The MHA Code gives guidance in relation to the treatment of young people and the admission and treatment of children.[15]

The MHA Code makes clear that young people with capacity can consent to their treatment[16] and those under 16 who are 'Gillick competent' can consent to admission and treatment.[17] In such cases, the child or young person's consent is sufficient authority for their informal admission and/or treatment. Significantly, the MHA Code advises against relying on parental consent where the child or young person refuses the proposed intervention. Noting that although in the past the courts have held that the refusal of a child or young person who is able to make relevant decision may be overridden by parental consent, thereby permitting the informal admission of a child or young person, in the light of the Human Rights Act 1998 and cases that 'reflect greater autonomy for competent under 18s', the MHA Code advises against relying on the consent of a person with parental responsibility.[18]

Children and young people unable to decide

If the child or young person is not able to make decisions about their admission and/or treatment, it may be possible for a person with parental responsibility to give the necessary consent, or in the case of young people the Mental Capacity Act 2005 (the MCA 2005)[19] may apply:[20]

> Young people and the MCA 2005: young people who lack capacity within the meaning of the MCA 2005 may be admitted to hospital and/or treated if such admission or treatment is in their best interests and does not amount to a 'deprivation of liberty' [discussed below on p. 201].
>
> Children and young people and 'the zone of parental control': Where the child is not able to make decisions about their admission and/or treatment, a person with parental responsibility may give the necessary consent if the proposed intervention falls within the 'zone of parental control'. Similarly, if the decision falls within the zone of parental control, parental consent may authorise the treatment of young people where they either lack capacity to make the treatment decision or are unable to do so because they are 'overwhelmed' [see below]. Parental consent may also authorise young people's admission to hospital where they lack capacity to make this decision.[21]

Zone of parental control

The 'zone of parental control' is a term used by the MHA Code to describe the basis for determining whether the proposed intervention can be authorised by the consent of a person with parental responsibility. It emphasises that there is a limit to the types of decisions that parents and others with parental responsibility are able to make on behalf of their children.

The MHA Code explains that there are no precise rules on what decisions are covered by the zone of parental control. Rather, each decision will need to be considered in the light of the particular circumstances of the case. The MHA Code suggests a range of factors that will be helpful to consider, such as the nature and invasiveness of the proposed intervention 'including the extent to which the child's liberty will be curtailed', the age and maturity of the child, whether the child is resisting and the extent to which the parent's interests may conflict with those of the child or the young person.[22]

Admission under the MHA 1983

As discussed above, if a child or young person is able to decide about admission to hospital and/or treatment but does not give their consent, practitioners can no longer rely on parental consent to authorise the proposed intervention. In order to proceed with the admission and/or treatment, consideration must be given as to whether the criteria for compulsory admission under the MHA 1983 are met.[23] Admission under the MHA 1983 will also need to be considered where:

- a child or young person is assessed as being unable to make the decision about admission and/or treatment but parental consent cannot be relied on because the relevant decision is outside the zone of parental control; or
- a young person lacks capacity but the MCA 2005 cannot be relied upon because the admission and/or treatment amounts to a deprivation of the young person's liberty.

If the criteria for detention under the MHA 1983 are not met, legal advice should be obtained on whether to seek a court order to authorise the proposed admission and/or treatment.

Detailed guidance on the assessment, and making applications, for detention in hospital under the MHA 1983, is set out in Chapter 4 of the MHA Code. The application is usually made by the Approved Mental Health Professional (AMHP)[24] and must be supported by two medical recommendations. However, where it is of urgent necessity for the person to be admitted and obtaining a second medical recommendation would cause undesirable delay, an application may be made on the basis of one medical recommendation (section 4 MHA 1983).

The MHA Code (36.51) states that treatment can be given without consent to a person aged under 18 if such treatment is necessary to 'preserve life or prevent irreversible serious deterioration of the patient's condition'. This is discussed in more detail in *The Legal Aspects of the Care and Treatment of Children and Young People with Mental Disorder: A Guide for Professionals.*[25] However, as Professor Phil Fennell notes, in relation to minors with mental disorder 'the circumstances in which emergency treatment without recourse to the Mental Health Act or the courts would be justified will surely be extremely exceptional'.[26]

The 'overwhelmed' young person

When considering the basis on which a young person is to be admitted to hospital and/or treated for their mental disorder, the starting point is that they are able to make such decisions for themselves.[27] If there are concerns that the young person is unable to make decisions about their admission to hospital and/or treatment, an assessment of their capacity should be undertaken in accordance with the MCA 2005, and the Code of Practice to the Mental Capacity Act 2005 (the MCA Code).

However, both the MHA Code and the MCA Code point to cases in which the young person is not able to make the relevant decision for reasons other than those prescribed by section 2 of the MCA 2005, namely due to an 'impairment of, or disturbance in the functioning of the mind or brain'. The Codes suggest that some young people may be unable to decide because they lack the maturity to do so, referring to such young people as 'being overwhelmed by the implications of the decision'.[28]

In most cases where admission to hospital and/or treatment for mental disorder is being considered, the cause of the young person's inability to make a decision is likely to be due to their mental disorder (in which case the MCA 2005 will apply). However, if a young person is too 'overwhelmed' to make the decision, rather than lacking capacity to do so (within the meaning of the MCA 2005), admission under the MHA 1983 will need to be considered. This is because the MCA 2005 is not applicable and parental consent cannot authorise the admission.[29]

Assessing Gillick competence for under 16s

Unlike the assessment of capacity, which is governed by the MCA 2005, with detailed guidance provided in the MCA Code, there is very little guidance on the assessment of under 16s. The MHA Code (36.38) states that a 'Gillick competent' child has a 'sufficient understanding and intelligence to enable them to understand fully what is involved in a proposed intervention'.

Although it is said to reflect the child's increasing development to maturity, the courts have also referred to the existence of a mental disorder as being relevant to Gillick competence. Reflecting this, the MHA Code advises that 'in some cases, for example because of a mental disorder, a child's mental state may fluctuate significantly' so that a child may appear to be competent to make a decision on some occasions but other times not able to do so. In such cases, practitioners are advised that 'careful consideration should be given to whether the child is truly Gillick competent at any time to take a relevant decision'.[30]

However, as Professor Fennell notes, the 'functional' aspects of decision making (i.e. the ability to decide) for Gillick competent children are similar to those under section 2 of the MCA 2005, for individuals aged 16 and over. For both age groups the issues considered cover understanding the information, retaining the information, weighing up such information to arrive at a decision and communicating that decision. The difference is that whereas with adults 'the functional incapacity must arise from an impairment of or disturbance in the functioning of the mind or brain', with children the inability to decide 'may arise from such a cause, but it could equally arise from immaturity or lack of intelligence'.[31] This is similar to the distinction made by the MHA Code between the young person who lacks capacity under the MCA 2005 and the 'overwhelmed' young person discussed above.

On this basis, when assessing the ability of under 16s to make decisions, it may be helpful to consider the impact of both the level of their maturity and understanding and their mental health problems on their ability to make the particular decision(s). Chapter 3 of the MCA Code provides guidance on helping people to make their own decisions.

The zone of parental control and deprivation of liberty

The relationship between the zone of parental authority and deprivation of liberty is unclear. For the reasons set out below, it is argued that if the restrictions placed on a child or young person amount to a deprivation of liberty, parental consent will not be sufficient authority for the proposed admission and/or treatment. In other words those with parental responsibility will not be able to consent to their child's deprivation of liberty because such a decision falls outside the zone of parental control. This view is at odds with the advice given in the MHA Code which suggests that in some circumstances parental consent may be able to authorise a child or young person's deprivation of liberty.[32] However, a recent decision (30 November 2011) of the Court of Appeal confirms that parents cannot authorise their child's detention:

> The decisions of the European Court of Human *Rights in Neilson* [sic] *v Denmark* [1998] 11EHRR 175 and of this court in *Re K* [2002] 2WLR 1141 demonstrate that an adult in the exercise of parental responsibility may impose, or may authorise others to impose, restrictions on the liberty of the child. However restrictions so imposed must not in their totality amount to detention. Detention engages the Article 5 rights of the child and a parent may not lawfully detain or authorise the detention of a child [emphasis added].[33]

In the light of the Court of Appeal's decision, before relying on parental consent to admit a child or young person informally, practitioners will need to give careful consideration as to whether the admission amounts to a deprivation of liberty.

Deprivation of liberty and Article 5 (the right to liberty)

There is no precise definition of 'deprivation of liberty'. The term derives from Article 5 of the European Convention on Human Rights which provides that everyone (including under 18s) has the right to liberty and individuals can only be deprived of their liberty in clearly prescribed circumstances. In establishing whether there is a deprivation of liberty it is necessary to consider all the circumstances of each case, looking at a range of factors such as the type, duration, effects and manner of implementation of the measure in question and the impact on the person concerned. It is unlikely that one single factor will, in itself, determine whether the overall set of steps being taken amount to a deprivation of liberty.[34]

The significance of finding that a person is deprived of their liberty was illustrated in *HL v United Kingdom*,[35] which concerned a man with learning disabilities who lacked capacity to agree to his admission to hospital and was admitted under the common law, in his best interests. Having concluded that he was deprived of his liberty, the European Court of Human Rights found that Mr L's rights under Article 5 had been breached. This is because while Article 5 permits the detention of individuals 'of unsound mind', this is only if the detention is 'in accordance with a procedure prescribed by law' (and the common law doctrine of necessity did not meet this requirement). Nor did Mr L have the opportunity to apply to a court to challenge the lawfulness of his detention as required by Article 5(4). Neither of these conditions is met in cases where children and young people are admitted to hospital and/or treated on the basis of parental consent. For example, the right to a review of their detention by a Mental Health Tribunal will not be available to them.

Limits to the scope of zone of parental control

The MHA Code refers to *Nielsen v Denmark*[36] as the main source of the concept of the zone of parental consent. This case was decided by the European Court of Human Rights over 20 years ago but despite the extensive case law in relation to adults since then, this remains the leading decision on the detention of under 18s. The Court held that the hospitalisation of a 12-year-old boy for over 5 months did not amount to a deprivation of liberty under Article 5 (as was claimed on behalf of the boy) but was the responsible exercise of the mother's custodial rights in the interests of her son.

This decision was subject to severe criticism for failing to give adequate protection to children's rights.[37] Arguably, in the light of the Convention on the Rights of the Child and more recent European Court of Human Rights cases, if a similar case were heard today it would be decided differently. For example, in a recent Supreme Court judgement, the decision in *Nielsen* was described as 'questionable' in so far as it relied on 'parental rights'.[38] Nonetheless, the following points will be relevant:

- There is a distinction between a restriction on a person's liberty and a deprivation of a person's liberty. Article 5 is only engaged if measures amount to a deprivation of liberty (although other rights such as Article 8 the right to private and family life must be respected).
- In *Nielsen v Denmark*, the European Court of Human Rights noted that the restrictions were not out of the ordinary for a boy of 12 who needed treatment in hospital, while the mother's actions were lawful and had a proper purpose.
- However, the Court acknowledged that the rights of the holder of parental authority are not unlimited and that it is incumbent on the State to provide safeguards from abuse.
- Indeed in a more recent case, the European Court of Rights emphasised that Article 5 places 'a positive obligation duty on the State to protect the liberty of it citizens'.[39]

In summary, while restrictions on a person's liberty do not engage Article 5 (so that parental consent may authorise appropriate restrictions), if the restrictions placed on a child or young person amount to a deprivation of liberty, Article 5 will be engaged and parental consent will not be sufficient authority for the proposed admission and/or treatment.

Rights in hospital

All children and young people should be informed of, and supported in exercising, their rights. Section 132 of the MHA 1983 requires hospital managers to ensure that detained patients are given information about their statutory rights both orally and in writing.[40] This includes being informed about the section of the MHA 1983 under which they are detained, what this means in practice (including the treatment provisions under Part 4 of the Act), and the right to apply to the Mental Health Tribunal. The MHA Code (2.45) states that informal patients should also be made aware of their legal position.

The following checklist highlights key areas to consider in relation to children and young people receiving inpatient care, in particular those who have been detained under the MHA 1983.

Rights in hospital – checklist

Provision of information about rights

- What arrangements have been made to provide children and young people with information about their rights?
- Is the information provided by people with sufficient training and experience of working with children and young people?
- Is the written information provided in an age-appropriate format?

The nearest relative

- Are children and young people who are detained under the MHA 1983 told who their nearest relative is, what role that person has under the MHA 1983 and, if the child or young person does not wish that person to be their nearest relative, the basis on which the nearest relative could be replaced?

Advocacy

- Are children and young people who are detained under the MHA 1983 informed about their right to be helped by an independent mental health advocate (IMHA) and supported in obtaining that help?[41]
- Are IMHAs trained to work with children and young people?
- What advocacy services are available for children and young people who are not detained?

Applying to the Mental Health Tribunal and/or hospital managers

- Are children and young people informed of their right to apply to the Mental Health Tribunal (and to be legally represented) and/or for a hospital managers' hearing for a review of their detention?
- What arrangements are in place to ensure that children and young people are assisted in applying to hospital managers' hearings and Mental Health Tribunals and are helped to obtain legal representation at an early stage?
- What arrangements are in place to notify the Mental Health Tribunal that the patient is aged under 18 and, in cases where the responsible clinician is not a CAMHS specialist, a CAMHS specialist prepares a report for the Tribunal.[42]

Care Quality Commission (CQC)

- Are children and young people informed when the CQC[43] is planning to visit the hospital, given an explanation of the role of the CQC and the right to meet privately with CQC representatives when they visit the hospital?

Consent to treatment

- Are children and young people informed about their rights in relation to consent to treatment, for example if they are detained under the MHA 1983, are they told about the circumstances in which they can be treated without their consent and the circumstances in which they have the right to refuse treatment?[44]

Involving the local authority

- What arrangements are in place to ensure that the relevant local authority is contacted:
  - When a child or young person who is subject to a care order or is 'looked after' is admitted to hospital?[45]
  - Where the child or young person is likely to be accommodated in hospital for three months or more (see sections 85 and 86 of the CA 1989 – the relevant local authority will be the one in which the child or young person has been living)?
  - iI the whereabouts of the person with parental responsibility is not known or that person has not visited the child for a considerable period of time?[46]

Complaints

- Are children and young people informed about their rights to make a complaint if they are not satisfied with aspects of their treatment or care (both under the hospital's complaints procedure and to the CQC) and how an advocate could assist them in pursuing such complaints?

Preparation for discharge

- What arrangements are in place to ensure that the child or young person's needs for aftercare services are undertaken in preparation for their discharge from hospital? (Chapter 4 of the *Transitions in Mental Health Care*[47] includes various case studies and checklists relevant to discharge planning.)

Compulsory powers in the community

The MHA 1983 includes provisions for the care and treatment of individuals living in the community, which may be relevant to children and young people receiving mental healthcare from Tier 4 CAMHS, namely section 17 leave, guardianship and supervised community treatment (SCT).

Children and young people who have been detained under the MHA 1983 may be given leave from hospital by the clinician with overall responsibility for the care of a patient detained under the Act (known as the 'Responsible Clinician') under section 17 of the Act. Guardianship may be applied to individuals aged 16 or over who have a 'mental disorder' and where the appointment of a guardian is considered necessary in the interests of the individual's welfare or for the protection of others. The purpose of guardianship is to enable individuals to receive care outside hospital when it cannot be provided without the use of compulsory powers.[48] The guardian can require i) the person to reside in a specified place, ii) the person to attend a specified place at specified times for medical treatment, occupation, education or training and iii) to be given access to the patient.[49]

Unlike guardianship, SCT can apply to individuals of all ages, including children and young people if the criteria for SCT are met. To be eligible for SCT a person must be detained in hospital under the MHA 1983 for treatment for their mental disorder (e.g. under Section 3 of the Act). SCT provides a framework for the management of patient care in the community and gives the responsible clinician the power to recall the patient to hospital for treatment if necessary.[50]

Further information on SCT, including the criteria for the use of SCT, the basis on which conditions can be imposed on those subject to SCT and how it applies to children and young people is provided in *The Legal Aspects of the Care and Treatment of Children and Young People with Mental Disorder: A Guide for Professionals*.[51] This guide suggests a number of points that might be useful to consider when deciding whether SCT is suitable for a child or young person. These are reflected in the checklist and Box 14.1.

Useful resources

The Mental Health Act 1983

Phil Fennell (2011) *Mental Health Law and Practice,* 2nd Edition, Jordans.
Richard Jones (2010) *Mental Health Act Manual,* 13th Edition, Sweet & Maxwell.
National Institute for Mental Health (2009) *The Legal Aspects of the Care and Treatment of Children and Young People with Mental Disorder: A Guide for Professionals,* January.
National Institute for Mental Health England (2008) *Supervised Community Treatment: A Guide for Practitioners,* October.

The Age-Appropriate Environment Duty

National Mental Health Development Unit (2009) *Working Together to Provide Age-Appropriate Environments and Services for Mental Health Patients Aged Under 18: A Briefing for Commissioners of Adult Mental Health Services and Child and Adolescent Mental Health Services,* June.
Camilla Parker (2010) *Responsibilities of NHS Trust Boards under Section 131A of the Mental Health Act 1983,* YoungMinds.

Community care

Steve Broach, Luke Clements, and Janet Read (2010) *Disabled Children: A Legal Handbook,* LAG & Council for Disabled Children (the full text is also online – see www.ncb.org.uk/cdc/resources/legal_handbook.aspx).

Luke Clements and Pauline Thompson (2007) *Community Care and the Law*, LAG, 5th Edition.
Camilla Parker with Luke Clements, Anthony Harbour and Jo Honigmann (2011) *Transitions in Mental Health Care – A Guide for Health and Social Care Professionals on the Legal Framework for the Care, Treatment and Support of Young People with Emotional and Psychological Problems During Their Transition Years*, YoungMinds, March.

BOX 14.1 Checklist: children and young people and SCT

Is the power to recall needed for this child or young person?
This is important because one of the conditions that must be met for SCT to be used is that the person can safely be treated for mental disorder in the community only if the responsible clinician has the power to recall the person to hospital for treatment should that be necessary.

Is the child or young person able and willing to consent to the treatment plan under SCT?
Although their consent to SCT is not required, in practice SCT patients will need to be involved in decisions about the treatment to be provided in the community and be prepared to cooperate with the proposed treatment (including the conditions attached to SCT). Furthermore, individuals who are subject to SCT and who have the capacity/competence to make decisions about their treatment cannot be given treatment without their consent. (Chapter 7 of The Legal Aspects of the Care and Treatment of Children and Young People with Mental Disorder: A Guide for Professionals explains the relevant provisions for treatment under SCT.)

What are the views of those with parental responsibility?
Those with parental responsibility may not consent (or refuse) treatment for mental disorder on behalf of their child who is subject to SCT. However, if a child or young person who is placed on SCT is living with one or both parents, the person giving the treatment should consult with the parent(s) about the particular treatment, given that the parent's objection would make it very difficult for the child or young person to live with their parents while on SCT.

Are those responsible for the child or young person willing and able to provide support?
It may be necessary to involve the patient's parent, or whoever will be responsible for looking after the child or young person, to ensure that they will be ready and able to provide the assistance and support that their child may need.

Notes

1 Department of Health, *Code of Practice, Mental Health Act 1983,* August 2008, London:TSO (referred to in this chapter as 'the MHA Code'). There is a separate Code of Practice for Wales, Welsh Assembly Government *Mental Health Code of Practice for Wales,* 2008, see: www.wales.nhs. uk/sites3/page.cfm?orgid=816&pid=33960. References in this chapter to the Code of Practice relate to the English MHA Code.

2 The Equality Act 2010 brings together the wide range of anti-discrimination legislation into one single Act. For further information see www.equalityhumanrights.com/legal-and-policy/ equality-act/

3 See MHA Code 36.78.

4 See MHA Code 36.6. The term 'parental responsibility' is defined in s3(1) Children Act 1989.

5 Department of Health, *Refocusing the Care Programme Approach: Policy and Positive Practice Guidance,* March 2008.

6 Camilla Parker with Luke Clements, Anthony Harbour and Jo Honigmann *Transitions in Mental Health Care – a guide for health and social care professionals on the legal framework for the care, treatment and support of young people with emotional and psychological problems during their transition years,* YoungMinds, March 2011.

7 See section 17 (10) and (110) of the CA 1989.

8 This term includes persons 'who suffer from mental disorder of any description'.

9 Section 117 of the Mental Health Act 1983 provides for the aftercare of certain patients who have been admitted to hospital under the MHA 1983, which will include all age groups.

10 See for example, Department of Health (2010) *Prioritising need in the context of Putting People First: a whole system approach to eligibility for social care – guidance on eligibility criteria for adult social care,* available at http://webarchive.nationalarchives.gov.uk/20130107105354/http://www.dh.gov.uk/prod_ consum_dh/groups/dh_digitalassets/@dh/@en/@ps/documents/digitalasset/dh_113155.pdf

11 For further information, see for example: Parker, C. (2010), *Age Appropriate Environment Duty: Section 131A Mental Health Act 1983 Commencement date 1st April 2010* Young Minds and O'Herlihy, A., et al (2009) *Aims SC4Y, Safe and Appropriate Care for Young People on Adult Mental Health Wards,* (2nd edition) available at http://www.rcpsych.ac.uk/PDF/AIMS-SC4Y%20) Standards%202009-2010.pdf

12 National Institute for Mental Health England, November 2009, available at: http://www. nmhdu.org.uk/silo/files/the-legal-aspects-of-the-care-and-treatment-of-children-and-young-- people.pdf

13 Available at: http://www.rcpsych.ac.uk/pdf/RT%20admission-to-hospital-and-treatment-for- mental-disorder-under-16s.pdf. Please note: the link incorrectly states that it concerns under 16s. Furthermore, in reference to the notes to this flow chart, the reader should be aware that since the publication of these flow charts, the courts have made clear that parents cannot authorise their child's deprivation of liberty – see below under the heading 'the zone of parental control and deprivation of liberty'.

14 http://www.rcpsych.ac.uk/pdf/RT%20admission-to-hospital-and-treatment-for-mental- disorder.pdf

15 MHA Code 36.21–36.50.

16 See section 8 of the Family Law Reform Act 1969.

17 This was established by *Gillick v West Norfolk and Wisbech Area Health Authority* [1986] A.C. 112.

18 See MHA Code 36.33 and 36.43.

19 Department of Constitutional Affairs, Mental Capacity Act 2005 Code of Practice, 2007 London: TSO.

20 Section 5 of the MCA 2005 permits decisions to be taken in connection with the care or treatment of a person who lacks capacity.

21 MHA Code 36.9.

22 MHA Code 36.12.

23 See sections 4, 2 and 3 of the MHA 1983. Chapter 4 of the MHA Code provides guidance on mental health assessments. See also *The Legal Aspects of the Care and Treatment of Children and Young People with Mental Disorder: A Guide for Professionals,* pages 44–46.

24 An application may also be made by the person's nearest relative but this is rare.
25 Page 59.
26 Phil Fennell, *Mental Health Law and Practice,* 2nd Edition, Jordans, 2011, 11.39.
27 This 'presumption of capacity' is set out in section 1(2) of the MCA 2005.
28 MHA Code 36.23.
29 The effect of section 131(2) of the MHA 1983 is that those with parental responsibility can only consent to the admission if the young person lacks capacity within the meaning of the MCA 2005.
30 MHA Code 36.40.
31 Phil Fennell, *Mental Health Law and Practice,* 2nd Edition, Jordans, 2011, 11.34.
32 See 36.25 and 36.26. See also the flow chart on page 352.
33 Re RK; *RK v BCC* [2011] EWCA Civ 1305.
34 Ministry of Justice, *Mental Capacity Act 2005, Deprivation of Liberty Safeguards, Code of Practice to supplement the main Mental Capacity Act 2005 Code of Practice*, August 2008, London: TSO. For a summary of recent cases on deprivation of liberty see: http://www.dh.gov.uk/en/SocialCare/Deliveringsocialcare/MentalCapacity/MentalCapacityActDeprivationofLibertySafeguards/index.htm. See *also Cheshire West & Chester Council v P* (2011) EWCA Civ 1257.
35 (Application 45508/99) (2004) 40 EHRR 761.
36 (1988) 11 EHRR 175.
37 See for example, David Feldman, *Civil Liberties and Human Rights in England and Wales*, Oxford University Press, 2nd edition, 2002, 459.
38 Lord Walker *Austin and another v Commissioner of Police of the Metropolis* [2009] UKHL 5, [2009] AC 564 at 45.
39 *Storck v Germany* (61603/00) 16th June 2005, 43 E.H.R.R. 6.
40 Section 132A of the Mental Health Act 1983 makes similar provisions relation to patients subject to supervised community treatment.
41 See Chapter 20 of the MHA Code for more information.
42 MHA Code 32.19.
43 The MHA Commission's functions have been transferred to the CQC.
44 See MHA Code 2.16.
45 Section 116 of the MHA 1983 (arranging visits etc.) and the MHA Code 36.80.
46 MHA Code 36.82.
47 See endnote 5.
48 MHA Code 26.2.
49 MHA 1983, section 8.
50 MHA Code 25.2–25.3.
51 See Chapter 6 (Supervised Community Treatment) and Chapter 7 (Treatment Regulated under Part 4A of the Mental Health Act 1983). See also National Institute for Mental Health England *Supervised Community Treatment: A Guide for Practitioners,* October 2008.

15

EDUCATION, TRAINING AND WORKFORCE DEVELOPMENT

Angela Sergeant

Key points

- Workforce development has been a major theme for health services and local authorities for much of the last decade. The quality of flexible staff, their availability both through supply and demand factors and overall value for money will be key factors in addressing future challenges.
- Alongside the policy and public agenda, the delivery of training and education is changing. Professional qualifications are now considered secondary to the competence and capability of the workforce.
- *Modernising Medical Careers* is transforming the way psychiatrists are trained. In response, a range of other enhanced roles such as specialist or advanced practitioner, some of which have a specific remit to include traditional medical roles, have been developed.
- Health Education England (HEE) and Local Education and Training Boards (LETBs) are required to work jointly to improve the quality of education and training outcomes so they meet the needs of service providers, patients and the public.
- Education and training departments will need to ensure that the workforce acquires leadership and business skills to lead change and meet the challenges of developing services. There is now a greater need to focus on income generation, tendering, project management, IT and e-learning.

Introduction

Modernising and strengthening the workforce is a central feature of current children's services and health policy. The vision for the children's workforce as described by the National CAMHS Support Service (NCSS, 2012) is a 'modern, skilled, competent, adaptable and flexible health, education and social care workforce providing a focused response to meet the needs of children and young people and their families'. Also, in terms of expectations, a 'better informed public' are demanding that clinicians show themselves to perform to higher standards than ever before.

We know that for children to have the best possible chances in life, when they come into contact with any child and mental health services, there needs to be a workforce that is respected by its peers and valued for the positive difference it makes to young people's lives. A workforce that is made up of people and volunteers that understand each other's roles can keep young people and children safer, make sure they flourish and help them overcome the barriers they face. To achieve this we must keep working together to increase the quality and capacity of the workforce (Children's Workforce Development Council, 2011) to deliver services in an integrated and effective way.

The overarching principle, that mental health is indeed 'everybody's business', continues to be a strong theme in the cross-government mental health outcomes strategy *No Health without Mental Health* (Department of Health, 2011).

> Tackling mental health problems early in life will improve educational attainment, employment opportunities and physical health, and reduce the levels of substance misuse, self-harm and suicide, as well as family conflict and social deprivation. Overall, it will increase life expectancy, economic productivity, social functioning and quality of life. It will also have benefits across the generations.
>
> (Royal College of Psychiatrists, 2010)

Alongside the influencing policy and public agenda, the delivery of training and education is changing. Professional qualifications are now considered secondary to the competence and capability of the workforce. The consideration of patient safety and improved clinical outcomes has led to the implementation of more workplace-based training and assessment. The Children's Workforce and Development Council (CWDC) acknowledge that in the current tighter fiscal climate, all services will need to work differently to reduce duplication, breaking silo working, and create consistency and cohesion across the workforce to face challenges in a cost-efficient and effective way (Children's Workforce Development Council, 2011).

It is important to take into account that the increasing influence and power of GP commissioning, greater patient choice and an increasing focus on outcomes suggests that workforce development will need to be systematically addressed in all areas if results are to be achieved at a time of reduced spending (National CAMHS Support Service, 2012). This chapter will discuss not only the influencing policies that affect the CAMHS workforce development but also the training and education implications. Finally, offering in conclusion the future direction of travel for the specialist CAMHS workforce.

Background and national guidance

According to the Children's Workforce and Development Council report (2011), the workforce is surprisingly diverse with more than 100 professions and occupations. The work is often delivered in small teams, typically not office-based and asked to deliver to target or task. They acknowledge that with the diversity of roles transforming practice across the workforce is a complex business. The CWDC will be investing in children's workforce development, with a total budget from the Department for Education of £113.4m, demonstrating the importance of continuing to support the people who work and volunteer with children, young people and families. They highlight that in the future the workforce will need to become more streamlined, as social enterprises and charities become more active in workforce development as they support local areas and employers to develop their staff.

There have been numerous reviews in the last few years that have noted the national changes in CAMHS and its impact on workforce development. In order to improve outcomes for children and young people The *National Service Framework for Children, Young People and Maternity Services* published back in 2004 by the Department of Health (2004a), set out its 10-year strategic plan for children's services which would ensure an adequately trained, motivated and resourced CAMHS workforce.

The *National Service Framework for Children, Young People and Maternity Services – Standard 9* (Department of Health, 2004a) identifies workforce related issues including:

- All staff working directly with children and young people have sufficient knowledge, training and support to promote the psychological well-being of children, young people and their families and to identify early indicators of difficulty.
- Arrangements are in place to ensure that specialist multidisciplinary teams (MDTs) are of sufficient size and have an appropriate skill mix, training and support to function effectively.

It places emphasis on people working with children and adolescents to have an understanding of child and adolescent mental health and skills.

The publication of *Every Child Matters* by the former Department for Education and Skills (DfES, 2003) highlighted that child mental health was 'everyone's business'. It endorsed the proposition that everyone working with children, young people and families should have a common set of skills and knowledge. Using *Every Child Matters* as a platform, the government set out to develop national occupational standards and a modular training and qualifications structure across the widest possible range of workers in children's services. This was to enable all people working with children to share a common core set of skills, knowledge and competence and help people move across professional boundaries. The Children's Workforce Unit was also tasked with increasing the availability of high quality continuous professional development for all adults who worked with children (DfES, 2003)

Building on these developments Nixon (2006) emphasised that in order to achieve good mental health in the nation's child population, all workers who come into contact with children, young people and their parents needed to have the educational opportunities to acquire the capabilities, knowledge, attitudes and skills, which will support children's mental health. The national CAMHS review (Department for Children, Schools and Families, 2008) upheld this recommendation and emphasised the need for CAMHS staff to enhance their specialist skills with a more comprehensive understanding of child development, mental health and psychological well-being. Furthermore it was acknowledged that local service commissioners and providers needed to ensure that their workforce was sufficient and skilled, well led and able to deliver high quality services. The CAMHS review suggested that the development of education and training opportunities would help commissioners shape a workforce in which specialist workers were trained, supervised and capable of delivering a full range of interventions based upon the best available evidence.

Workforce issues

The Royal College of Psychiatrists (2006) suggests that Tier 4 workforce planning and training must be addressed on a regional level and a workforce plan drawn up concomitantly with business plans for new services. Workforce planning and development is a dynamic process which evolves over time as priorities, processes and capabilities develop and change. Workforce development has been a major theme for health services and local authorities for much of the last decade. High quality services for mental health and emotional well-being rely on committed staff in many different sectors, working in new and innovative ways, suggest the National CAMHS Support Service (2012) and, therefore, planning and developing the workforce effectively is the foundation for such change. This can help meet the goal of having the right people, in the right place, working to their capabilities and with those capabilities matched to the needs of service users.

In setting out its vision through the *National Service Framework for Children, Young People and Maternity Services* the Department of Health (2004a) poses a serious challenge to create a workforce of sufficient numbers with the right capabilities across all professional and non-professionally affiliated groups. The NSF states that 'providing high quality CAMHS is dependent on having sufficient numbers of appropriately trained staff to deliver high quality services in all four tiers, with a balanced skill mix to ensure the necessary range of skills'. The NSF goes on to state that the provision of mental healthcare for children and young people and their families can be emotionally demanding and stressful, particularly where there are high levels of risk. As such, the NSF stated that support systems to enable staff to practice effectively and safely include the availability of supervision, appraisal, continuing professional development (CPD) and mentoring. This is in the context of clear clinical and supervisory arrangements and structures in place for all staff to ensure accountable and safe service delivery (Department of Health, 2004a).

The Centre for Workforce Intelligence (CFWI) established a 'horizon scanning capability' and set out the programme for 2012–2013 to inform strategic planning on the configuration of roles, skills and competencies across the public sector. It identified big picture challenges facing health and social care such as 'reforming medical training', creating a flexible workforce, uncertainty over funding whilst improving efficiency and productivity (Centre for Workforce Intelligence, 2012).

Current financial pressures and the Quality, Innovation, Productivity and Prevention (QIPP) agenda are driving organisations to plan more strategically. The quality of flexible staff, their availability both through supply and demand factors and overall value for money will be key factors in addressing this challenge. The modernisation agenda for CAMHS and children's services generally envisaged substantial growth and change (although in recent years most services have been the subject of staff skill mix review, in order to manage

BOX 15.1   Understanding workforce issues

1   improving workforce design and planning so as to root it in local service planning and delivery;
2   identifying and using creative means to recruit and retain people in the workforce;
3   facilitating new ways of working across professional boundaries;
4   creating new roles to tap into a new recruitment pool and so complement existing staff types;
5   developing the workforce through revised education and training at both pre- and post-qualification levels;
6   developing leadership and change management skills.

Source: Adapted from Nixon (2006).

cost improvement plans (CIP) savings. According to Nixon (2006), the implementation of national guidance with its associated investment has in the past been hindered by the difficulties in recruitment and retaining appropriately trained staff.

This situation may continue as services are constantly forced to review their skill mix to achieve financial goals and adhere to evidence-based interventions. With this in mind there appears to be a realignment of staff returning to their professional 'core business', for example with psychiatrists only seeing the most severe, complex children and young people or those for whom detention under the Mental Health Act is being considered.

In *Understanding Workforce Issues in CAMHS* (Nixon, 2006) identified six key themes to be addressed considered by workforce planners (see Box 15.1).

With the increased establishment of home treatment teams and early intervention services in child and adolescent services, it is clear that the type of work carried out by Tier 4 CAMHS nowadays is much more complex and challenging than ever before. An adequate and competent workforce is fundamental to improving outcomes for children and young people.

Some professionals entering specialist posts within CAMHS do not hold specific child and adolescent qualifications and in some cases have not worked within a child and adolescent environment. In many areas there is a lack of advanced training programmes for professionals working directly with children and young people, and this could have a major impact on the type of services provided to many children, young people and families (Nixon, 2006). Kurtz (2009) adds to the concerns regarding the specialist CAMHS workforce by identifying that there is a lack of training in children's mental health for most professional's core training and more advanced training programmes for working directly with children and young people.

Tier 4 services are only one part of comprehensive CAMHS and the interventions offered need to be safe, timely and effective and able to respond to the wide range of needs which include the provision of: specialist and multidisciplinary assessment and treatment services; teaching, specialist consultation and liaison services; research and audit; and support, training and consultation.

Therefore a variety of therapeutic skills are needed, including behavioural, cognitive, interpersonal/psychodynamic, pharmacological and systemic approaches. These skills are not necessarily all vested in particular disciplines so that a combination of a skills-based and professional-based approach to team development is appropriate.

The workforce skills required within inpatient treatment in the future are likely to be very different with changes to Tier 4 core business and ethos. For example the impact of shorter inpatient stays will require service providers to review the skill set. Kurtz (2009) highlights the development of intensive community teams which will alter the focus of inpatient treatment, with increasing emphasis on symptom stabilisation and minimum necessary change before rapid discharge of the client. Collaborative workforce planning across the tiers will be crucial in preparing a specialist workforce supporting this change and requires coordinated financing, commissioning and delivery of appropriate training and education.

New ways of working

Nearly every intervention set out in *Every Child Matters* and the children's NSF has implications for the children's workforce. In order to improve outcomes for children and young people there needs to be an adequately resourced, trained and motivated workforce.

New ways of working (NWW) in mental health has been evolving since 2003 and the CAMHS specific component started in 2006. The aim of the CAMHS project was to look across professions as well as within professions. The introduction of NWW challenged professionals to be more flexible and take on wider roles than their traditional training would have enabled them to do. NWW has been a major force for work reform since it began back in 2003. Although it started with psychiatrists, it has subsequently been embraced by all professional bodies representing nurse, social workers, applied psychologists and other health professionals (Department of Health, 2007).

The overall aim of NWW has been to:

> Make the best of scarce clinical resources: to enable those staff with the most expertise and skills to work with those with the most complex needs; and to supervise and develop other staff to extend their roles and competence to undertake work previously undertaken by people working at consultant level. This requires professionals to explore new ways of working and the development of new roles within CAMHS to better meet the needs of children and young people.

The New Ways of Working Programme encouraged the development of new, enhanced and changed roles, and the redesign of systems and processes to support staff to deliver effective, person-centred care in a way that is personally, financially and organisationally sustainable. It recognised that cultural change lies at the heart of any kind of workforce reform, as it involves rethinking established values, ways of working and roles. Though the programme itself has come to an end, the approach remains central to workforce planning and development.

Moving from a workforce defined and restricted by professional qualifications to one defined by skills, competencies and capability can be challenging for the current workforce and has implications for the training and development of future staff (Morris and Nixon, 2008).

The National CAMHS Workforce Programme supported by the National CAMHS Workforce Subgroup commissioned a project in 2007 exploring new ways of working in CAMHS. The project concluded that, in view of the ageing healthcare workforce, there was a need to concentrate on staff development to ensure that the future CAMHS workforce has the appropriate mix of skills and competencies to meet the needs of the population it serves. It recommended that in addition to generic skills, CAMHS workers should be trained, supervised and supported to be capable of delivering a full range of specialist interventions, based upon the best available evidence.

The philosophy of the new ways of working approach was: 'using the skills, knowledge and experience of consultant psychiatrists to best effect by concentrating on service users with the most complex needs, acting as a consultant to MDTs, promoting distributed responsibility and leadership across teams to achieve a cultural shift in services' (Care Services Improvement Partnership et al., 2005, p. 5). Consultants should have a smaller caseload of patients with whom they are able to exercise their competences directly. This should, in turn, mean a redistribution of tasks around the members of the MDT on the basis of interest, skills and experience rather than discipline of origin, with doctors acting as consultant to them in the broadest sense of the word. These are exactly the principles behind the NWW projects in mental health.

Indeed changes are currently underway within CAMHS as consultants and their medical colleagues change their practices. It is not possible to make a change to one staff group without having an impact on the rest of the workforce and one change that has had a significant impact on the medical profession is the introduction of the European Working Time Directive for doctors. This placed strict limits on the hours junior doctors can work, resulting in a rethink of the traditional medical roles. *Modernising Medical Careers* (Department of Health, 2004b) influenced future training roles for consultants and in 2004 a new contract for consultants was introduced for the first time since the inception of the NHS. This is already having an impact in the way consultant psychiatrists undertake their roles within CAMHS teams. There is reducing ambiguity about consultants' roles, with an increasingly clear expectation that they provide clinical leadership, and function as a generic member of the MDT. This is not just true for medical consultants, but also nurse and psychology consultants.

These issues have been revisited through the creating capable teams approach, developed as part of the New Ways of Working programme (Department of Health, 2007). In some areas, trusts are employing specialist nurses as part of a medical team to take on traditionally medical roles such as medication histories and physical reviews. This team approach is likely to be of increasing importance as changes in junior doctors' working hours and training make it more difficult for them to ensure continuity of care in a ward setting.

The updated mental health legislation in England (the Mental Health Act, 2007) offers the opportunity to extend the responsible clinician (RC) role to other professional groups.

However, the extent to which these responsibilities will be welcomed or taken up by others is not yet clear. *Modernising Medical Careers* will also transform the way psychiatrists are trained. In response, many areas have developed a range of other enhanced roles such as specialist or advanced practitioner, some of which have a specific remit to include traditional medical roles. One example of extended roles is non-medical prescribing; currently open to nurses and pharmacists (National Prescribing Centre et al., 2005). With the appropriate training and qualification, non-medical prescribers can now prescribe the full range of medications, through either independent or supplementary prescribing (Brimblecombe et al., 2005).

The disadvantages of strict adherence to traditional professional groupings are becoming more apparent and are exemplified by the blurring of roles for many professionals. Professional bodies can be protective of their current boundaries and practice and staff may fear that their professional roles will change. Consideration of potential new roles within CAMHS offers scope to fill identified gaps in the service with a practitioner with the required skills rather than by a particular professional grouping. With the publication of *No Health without Mental Health* (Department of Health, 2011) there is a plan to expand the front line workforce and review the contribution that professionals make to develop the mental health of children and young people.

Education and training

Education and training need to be responsive to the skills and competencies required for healthcare delivery. It is critically important that the needs of patients for care, and of the NHS and others as providers of care, drive the education and training agenda. The policy framework for a new approach to workforce planning and the education and training of the health workforce, *Liberating the NHS: Developing the Healthcare Workforce – From Design to Delivery* (Department of Health, 2012), sets out its plan to reform the education and training system to improve care and outcomes for patients. It aims to provide a better educational experience for trainees to attain the right professional and clinical skills that enable health workers to adapt quickly to innovation in service models.

There are two central planks to the new system – Health Education England (HEE) and the Local Education and Training Boards (LETBs) – that will work together to improve the quality of education and training outcomes so they meet the needs of service providers, patients and the public plus drive up the quality of the workforce to provide better outcomes and health improvement.

Turning attention to Tier 4 CAMHS, the reality is that attendance at training is an ongoing issue for Tier 4 CAMHS staff. There are still barriers to accessing training, notably a lack of training budget and/or a lack of staff cover to enable CAMHS staff members to attend training sessions. The Quality Network for Inpatient CAMHS (QNIC, 2007) highlighted that whilst provision and ability to attend training had improved somewhat, access to training was still an issue. The report notes that the individuals who could benefit most from undertaking training sessions, tended to be those that were the most difficult to release from ward duties, i.e. registered and unregistered nursing staff. On a more positive note, the report confirmed that CAMHS inpatient units usually adhered to

BOX 15.2   Tier 4 CAMHS training

Assessments including risk assessment and management

- safeguarding and promoting the welfare of children;
- care co-ordination including transfer of care;
- managing relationships and boundaries between young people and staff, including appropriate touch;
- use of formal observations;
- consent and capacity;
- legal frameworks such as the Children Acts, Mental Health Act 2007, the revised Code of Practice, Disability Discrimination Act and The Mental Capacity Act 2005
- Resuscitation (child and adult);
- management of imminent and actual violence, breakaway techniques and restraint measures;
- audit and research skills;
- staff receive training on the evidence underpinning the range of treatments provided for example, NICE guidelines, 'Drawing on the Evidence' – Wolpert et al., 2006.

Source: QNIC (2012)

specific mandatory training for all staff and a locally delivered, annual training plan. Most services have an in-house induction and training programme.

In 2012 QNIC published its latest recommendations for core staff training in Tier 4 CAMHS (see Box 15.2).

The CAMHS review (Department for Children, Schools and Families, 2008) highlighted that the staff with the least experience of mental health issues are often the ones who spend the majority of time with the most vulnerable children. This is especially the case in Tier 4 units, which frequently have a heavy reliance on bank and/or agency staff, or a high proportion of healthcare support workers within their workforce.

In the report written by Kurtz (2007) from a review of Tier 4 CAMHS in the nine regions of England, there was recognition that the dividing line between Tier 4 and Tier 3 is essentially unclear and there is no way to make a clear distinction that is generalisable across the whole country. The findings also suggest an implicit notion that the admission criteria in CAMHS inpatient units may often be based upon the perceived capability of the staff working within that setting and their related skill set. The report raised concerns regarding the lack of staff supervision and access to specialist in-house training during challenging periods. It was apparent that poor staff development, competence and confidence to deal with complex cases had a negative impact upon the retention of staff. It stresses the need for reflective opportunities, consultation with relevant others and appropriate supervision of their work.

Recruitment and retention is a significant challenge, especially for Tier 4 inpatient units and there is a constant need to consider offering more flexible entry routes and building more rewarding careers which will help to ensure retention of staff. The drain of staff from inpatient CAMHS to community settings is an important workforce issue that is familiar to CAMHS service providers and commissioners (O'Herlihy et al., 1999). One traditionally held view is that individuals spend a couple of years to 'get the basics' in CAMHS before moving onto better opportunities in CAMHS community settings. It is fair to say that inpatient units have struggled to evidence that they provide a supportive professional learning environment. However, this perception is changing and should continue to alter. In recent years inpatient CAMHS has demonstrated an eagerness to develop national benchmarks in standards of care and compliance with these standards. With the development of a Quality Network for Inpatient CAMHS (QNIC) inpatient units have embraced the opportunity to open their doors to external review and to learn from feedback and advice. They have been able to prove evidence of considerable improvements year on year in their annual reports.

The workplace learning environment is crucial to maintain a dynamic service that is not only an attractive career opportunity but has the ability to retain clinical expertise. The national CAMHS review final report (Department for Children, Schools and Families, 2008) offered key recommendations regarding training and development for the people who work with young people. These seek to ensure that there is an improved basic knowledge of child development, mental health and psychological well-being across the children's workforce.

If the culture, within the CAMHS inpatient setting, continues to encourage gaining and sharing knowledge, this may lift morale, improve clinical care and positively benefit staff retention. The ultimate goal is to boost service delivery, improve standards of patient care, improve clinical outcomes and enhance the reputation of the unit, which would benefit staff members and reassure patients and their families.

One approach to creating a positive learning environment is the development of a dynamic learning culture. Key principles that apply to developing a dynamic learning culture according to NHS Education South Central (2009) are as follows:

- allow trainers and trainees time for reflection and study activities;
- encourage experienced educators to share the benefits of supporting learners with others in the team;
- develop buddy systems for new staff and be supportive of new staff;
- participate in induction programmes;
- develop education materials;
- share good practice;
- develop an 'education notice board';
- develop inter-professional learning activities.

Strong leadership, management and supportive commissioning alongside the development of new models of practice will be required to sustain a professional learning environment within Tier 4 services. Training staff should be a high priority, as is the retention of existing staff and recruiting staff, and ensuring that staff members and teams are provided with appropriate and timely learning opportunities. Training should be linked to appraisals and service requirements. Good role modelling, within clinical practice areas, may reinforce good standards of care and assist in developing an atmosphere of enquiry and learning.

In order to make best use of the highly trained professionals in CAMHS it is essential to support them to work most effectively and efficiently. We must explore new roles to complement service model changes and create career pathways so that a Tier 4 service is not only an attractive career opportunity but has the ability to retain clinical expertise. If there is closer interplay between Tier 3 and Tier 4 services, training opportunities should be considered across inpatient, day patient and outpatient CAMHS and skills enhanced by using rotational or across-tier employment opportunities.

It will be crucial for the future to ensure that commissioned child and adolescent mental health education and training programmes include an objective rating of quality in relation to their relevance to the implementation of the modernisation agenda for children's services across all sectors, and specific CAMHS policy will be crucial in the future (Department of Health, 2004a; 2004d). According to *No Health Without Mental Health* (Department of Health, 2011), another important factor for education, training and the quality of service delivery will be introduction of Payment by Results for children's mental health services, to improve outcomes and incentives for CAMHS and focus the minds of providers.

Core competency training

An essential element of ensuring quality services for children and young people is that future education and training available to the workforce meets the demands of the new developments in children's services. *Everybody's Business* (Department of Health, 2001) highlights that the needs of children and young people are different from those of adults, therefore CAMHS staff will require particular skills and knowledge to meet these needs. Despite this, much of the core professionals' education curriculum does not to include child and adolescent mental health in its pre-registration training.

A key strategic component to workforce redesign has been the development and use of competencies. Competencies are descriptors of the performance criteria, knowledge and understanding that are required to undertake work activity. According to NHS Education for Scotland 2011, there is a clear professional consensus that interventions in CAMHS rest on a set of 'underpinning' skills (core and generic therapeutic competencies) as well as a set of assessment skills. This document highlights the need for the competencies to be of practical use, that accurately represent the approach both as a theoretical model and in terms of its clinical application.

There have been a number of influential documents/papers recommending the development of core skills and competencies across disciplines, such as *New Ways of Working* (Department of Health, 2007), the *Creating Capable Teams Approach* (Department of Health, 2007) and the *Knowledge and Skills Framework* (Department of Health, 2004e). This has allowed services to think creatively and build a workforce that can be measured by quality standards not just by the professional qualifications of the staff. *Delivering Workforce Capacity, Capability and Sustainability in Child and Adolescent Mental Health Services* (Nixon, 2006) seeks to ensure that the skills and competencies of the CAMHS workforce at all levels of service provision meet the mental health needs of the population served. In addition to the generic skills required it also recommends that specialist workers should be trained, supervised and supported to be capable of delivering a full range of interventions, based upon the best available evidence.

The Knowledge and Skills Framework (Department of Health, 2004b) links practice closely with education and training and identifies how education and training has evolved to ensure practice is developed through competency frameworks. These aim to increase the capability and effectiveness of the workforce linking the *Common Core Skills and Knowledge for the Children's Workforce* (Department of Education and Skills, 2005); the national occupational standards (Care Services Improvement Partnership & National Institute for Mental Health in England, 2007) and the *Ten Essential Shared Capabilities* (Department of Health, 2004c) altogether.

With the establishment of Skills for Health, *Core Functions: Child and Adolescent Mental Health Services, Tiers 3 & 4* (Skills for Health, 2007) and the *Common Core of Skills and Knowledge* (Children's Workforce Development Council, 2010) were developed. Within these documents, key areas of expertise were identified in which any CAMHS worker should be able to demonstrate their competency. The *Common Core of Skills and Knowledge for the Children's Workforce* describes the skills and knowledge that everyone who works with children and young people (including volunteers) is expected to have. The six areas of expertise offer a single framework to underpin multi-agency and integrated working, professional standards, training and qualifications across the children's workforce (Children's Workforce Development Council, 2010).

These competencies describe what CAMHS staff members need to do and to know in order to carry out this activity, regardless of who performs it. The common core describes the skills and knowledge that everyone who works with children and young people is expected to have. It reflects a set of common values for practitioners and recognises that some roles will place greater emphasis on one of more of the common core headings. These functions are as follows;

- effective communication and engagement with children, young people, their families and carers;
- assessment;
- safeguarding and promoting the welfare of children;
- care coordination;
- promoting health and well-being;
- supporting transitions;
- multi-agency working;
- sharing information;
- professional development and learning.

In addition to these functions, it is important to acknowledge that each particular discipline brings its own perspective, based on theoretical models and underpinning principles. The MDT working of specialist CAMHS is a key aspect of its functioning, using evidence-based practice approaches, and embracing and utilising diverse approaches, whilst finding synergy between different theoretical models that brings richness to the assessment and treatment of children and young people with mental health problems. The Department of Health intends to work with the Royal College of Nursing to examine the skills and competencies required of CAMHS nurses (McDougall, 2011). Many local areas are already using the common core effectively in induction, training, job descriptions and workforce development strategies.

Education and training has to be seen in the context of CPD. The notion of CPD is based on the idea that we need to be engaged in lifelong learning. The learning we had in the past and our current understanding will be helpful and make a significant contribution to the work we complete. This should be linked to an annual review/ appraisal system setting out clear objectives for future training needs and linked to the training needs analysis of the service. Delivery of training is always evolving and needs to make best use of available technologies. There is increasing need to digitalise delivery of learning and information, and join up information, providing it in a format that makes sense to all staff.

Education and training departments will need to ensure that the workforce acquire leadership and business skills to lead change and meet the challenges of developing the core business, including income generation, tendering, project management, IT and the increased use of training via e-learning.

A Tier 4 practitioner's handbook

Recognising that workforce in Tier 4 inpatient CAMHS needed access to better education and training resources, the NCSS commissioned the development of guidance for staff working in these services. A practitioner's handbook was developed by the author (Department of Health, 2009) which focused on the five following key areas:

1   child, adolescent and family development;
2   role and function of inpatient CAMHS practitioner;
3   staff support and well-being;
4   risk management;
5   the inpatient pathway.

Using the practitioner's handbook as a reference point, an online learning resource (http://in-patienttraining.camhs.org.uk/) encourages inpatient staff to interact with the ideas by questioning, evaluating and reflecting to enhance their learning experience.

Clinical supervision

Clinical supervision presents a crucial opportunity for professional support and learning to explore the valuable elements of clinical practice. It is excellent practice to encourage reflection within supervision to support learning processes. Clinical supervision allows the practitioner to reflect on their interactions and examine everyday situations in a supportive manner. Reflective practice should be a fundamental part of the working lives of CAMHS inpatient staff members to help prevent burnout and professional complacency.

The Department of Health (1993) document *A Vision for the Future* defines clinical supervision as:

> a formal process of professional support and learning, which enables individual practitioners to develop knowledge and competence, assume responsibility for their own practice and enhance consumer protection and the safety of care in clinical situations... central to the process of learning and to the expansion of the scope of practice... encouraging self assessment and analytical and reflective skills.
>
> (Royal College of Nursing, 2003).

Clinical supervision and reflective practice present crucial learning opportunities for professionals to explore the valuable elements of practice and to promote professional development, for example through learning action plans. Supervision may be delivered on a one-to-one basis and its nature may be clinical, managerial and/or educational. Finding time to explore problems, difficulties and feelings encountered within inpatient CAMHS work is crucially important. Supervision is one mechanism which may be used and a group supervision format may facilitate the inpatient team to reflect and to discuss pertinent issues. Supervision may enable the professional to become more self-assured and grow in confidence and to broaden his/her thinking through problem solving.

The future for specialist CAMHS

In the coming years, workforce development and planning will be a key vehicle for providing continued improvement in quality and productivity to deliver the best possible outcomes for the local population. Simply doing the same things in the same way, argue the NCSS (2012), is unlikely to deliver the vision of ensuring a world-class children and young people's workforce. They conclude that finding creative and innovative ways of working will require significant change, but if successful will have a considerable impact.

As Nixon back in 2006 highlighted, some questions that have vexed professionals for years will probably continue: for example should specialist CAMHS sit within children's services, or mental health services, or can CAMHS straddle both? Will the investment in universal services and early intervention be matched by better funding for secondary and tertiary care for child and adolescent mental health? Should there be an entirely new conception of CAMHS, sitting within integrated child and youth services? And, finally, what will the future CAMHS workforce look like?

Having effective leadership in place at all levels across all agencies is crucial to facilitating the engagement of both staff and organisations in modernising CAMHS. Successful leadership in CAMHS means the ability to bring about and sustain new models of service and to improve the overall mental health of children and young people. The key strategic documents need to be translated into the local context, ensuring that all parties are signed up to the key challenges. As the Field Review (2010) (cited in the *Centre for Social Justice, 2011*) acknowledges: 'important changes can and do take place later in children's lives and…investment in the early years will not be fully effective unless it is followed up with high quality services for those who need them most later in childhood'.

The impact of the Health and Social Care Act (2012) will significantly change the health and social care landscape (NCSS, 2012) and the mental health strategy will further develop this, with CAMHS finding themselves with new commissioners and changed priorities. There will be a clear need for strong leadership and leaders in CAMHS, guiding children's emotional health, well-being and mental health through this process. Leadership capacity in CAMHS will be required to deliver better outcomes for children and young people and the quality of CAMHS staff will be integral to achieving this. Employers now use the internet as a key source of information, advice and guidance, but continue to value the importance of local networks and forums. They like to access more 'relevant' information in order to 'make informed choices' and to be able to better see the links between local, regional and national practice (Children's Workforce Development Council, 2011).

The government is likely to increase the numbers and improve the skills of those working in priority areas, such as early years, children, young peoples' families social work and educational psychology but will stop centrally funding programmes and expect employers and professionals to take greater responsibility for training and development themselves (Children's Workforce Development Council, 2011). Therefore all services will need to move closer to the vision of a united workforce which comes together to provide support and services that meet the needs of children, young people and families whist demonstrating their cost-effectiveness and high quality provision.

References

Brimblecombe, N., Parr, A. & Gray, R. (2005) Medication and mental health nurses: developing new ways of working, *Mental Health Practice*, 8(5), 12–14.

Care Services Improvement Partnership, National Institute for Mental Health in England, Changing Workforce Programme & Royal College of Psychiatrists. (2005) *New Ways of Working for Psychiatrists: Enhancing Effective, Person-Centred Services through New Ways of Working in Multidisciplinary and Multi-Agency Contexts. Final Report 'But Not the End of the Story'.* London: DH.

Centre for Social Justice (2011) *Outcome- based Government.* London: Centre for Social Justice.

Centre for Workforce Intelligence. (2012) *Workforce Planning Along Care Pathways: The CFWI Care Pathways Toolkit.* London: CWFI.

Children's Workforce Development Council. (2010) *Common Core of Skills and Knowledge for the Children's Workforce.* London: Department of Education and Skills.

Children's Workforce Development Council. (2011) *Children's Workforce Matters: Business Plan 2011/2012.* Leeds. www.cwdcouncil.org.uk

Department for Children, Schools and Families. (2008) *Children and Young People in Mind: The Final Report of the National CAMHS Review.* London: HMSO.

Department for Education and Skills. (2003) *Every Child Matters – Summary.* London: HMSO.

Department for Education and Skills. (2005) *Common Core Skills and Knowledge for the Children's Workforce.* London: DfES.

Department of Health. (1993) *A Vision for the Future: Report of the Chief Nursing Officer.* London: HMSO.

Department of Health. (2001) *Everybody's Business: Integrated Mental Health Services for Older Adults: A Service Development Guide.* Leeds: Care Services Improvement Programme (CSIP).

Department of Health. (2004a) *National Service Framework for Children, Young People and Maternity Services – Standard 9: The Mental Health and Psychological Well-being of Children and Young People.* London: DH.

Department of Health. (2004b) *Modernising Medical Careers: The Next Steps. The Future Shape of Foundation, Specialist and General Practice Training Programmes.* London: DH.

Department of Health. (2004c) *Ten Essential Shared Capabilities*. London: DH.

Department of Health. (2004d) *Getting the Right Start: National Service Framework for Children Emerging Findings*. London: DH.

Department of Health. (2004e) *The NHS Knowledge and Skills Framework (NHS KSF) and the Development Review Process*. London: DH.

Department of Health. (2007) *Creating Capable Teams Approach: Best Practice Guidance to Support the Implementation of New Ways of Working and New Roles*. London: DH.

Department of Health. (2009) *Working within Child and Adolescent Inpatient Services: A Practitioner's Handbook by Angela Sergeant*. London: NCSS.

Department of Health. (2011) *No Health without Mental Health*. London: DH.

Department of Health. (2012) *Liberating the NHS: Developing the Healthcare Workforce – From Design to Delivery*. London: DH.

Field, F. (2010) *The Foundation Years: preventing poor children becoming poor adults*. London: The Stationery Office.

Kurtz, K. (2009) *The Evidence Base to Guide Development of Tier 4 CAMHS*. London: DH.

Kurtz, Z. (2007) *Regional Reviews of Tier 4 Child and Adolescent Mental Health Services: Summary and Comment*. Leicester: Care Services Improvement Partnership (CSIP)/National CAMHS Support Service.

McDougall, T. (2011) Mental health problems in childhood and adolescence. *Nursing Standard* 26(14): 48–56.

Morris, T. & Nixon, B. (2008) New ways of working in CAMHS. *The Journal of Mental Health Training, Education and Practice*, 3, 22–27.

National CAMHS Support Service. (2012) *Better Mental Health Outcomes for Children and Young People*. www.chimat.org.uk/camhs/commissioning.

National Prescribing Centre, National Institute for Mental Health in England & Department of Health. (2005) *Improving Mental Health Services by Extending the Role of Nurses in Prescribing and Supplying Medication: Good Practice Guide*. London: NPC, NIHME & Department of Health.

NHS Education for Scotland. (2011) *Core competency framework for the protection of children*. Edinburgh: NMS Scotland.

NHS Education South Central. (2009) *Supporting Learning and Development Across NHS South Central*. Spring Edition. Southampton: NESC Education.

Nixon, B. (2004) Towards an Understanding of Workforce Issues in CAMHS. In *Understanding Workforce Issues in CAMHS: Conference Handbook*. Report to National CAMHS Support Service. London: National CAMHS Support Service.

Nixon, B. (2006) *Delivering Workforce Capacity, Capability and Sustainability in Child and Adolescent Mental Health Services*. London: Care Services Improvement Programme (CSIP).

O'Herlihy, A., Worrall, A., Banerjee S., Jaffa, T., Mears, P., Brook, H., Scott, A., White, R., Nikolaou, V. & Lelliot, P. (1999) *National Inpatient Child and Adolescent Psychiatry Study (NICAPS). Initial Report to the Department of Health*. London: Royal College of Psychiatrists' Research Unit.

QNIC (2007) *QNIC Annual Report – Quality Network for Inpatient CAMHS:* London: Royal College of Psychiatrists' Research Unit.

QNIC (2012) *QNIC Annual Report- Quality Network for Inpatient CAMHS*. London: Royal College of Psychiatrists' Research Unit.

Royal College of Nursing. (2003) *Clinical Supervision in the Workplace*. London: RCN.

Royal College of Psychiatrists. (2006) *Roles and Responsibilities of the Consultant in General Adult Psychiatry* (Council Report CR140). London: Royal College of Psychiatrists.

The Centre for Social Justice. (2011) *Making Sense of Early Intervention: A Framework for Professionals*. London: Centre for Social Justice.

Wolpert, M., Fuggle, P., Cottrell, D., Fonagy, P., Phillips, J., Pilling, S., Stein, S. & Target, M. (2006) *Drawing on the Evidence. Advice for Mental Health Professionals Working with Children and Adolescents*. London: CAMHS Publications.

INDEX

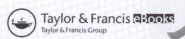